A Social History of Maternity and Childbirth

People are fascinated by stories of childbirth, and the sources to document maternity in Britain in the twentieth century are rich and varied. This book puts the history of maternity in England into its wider social context, highlighting areas of change and continuity, and charting the development of pregnancy and birth as it emerged from the shadows and became central to social debate.

A Social History of Maternity and Childbirth considers the significance of the regulation and training of midwives and doctors, exploring important aspects of maternity care including efforts to tackle maternal deaths, the move of birth from home to hospital, and the rise of consumer groups. Using oral histories and women's memoirs, as well as local health records and contemporary reports and papers, this book explores the experiences of women and families, and includes the voices of women, midwives and doctors. Key themes are discussed throughout, including:

- the work and status of the midwife
- the place of birth
- pain relief
- ante- and postnatal care
- women's pressure groups
- high-tech versus low-tech
- political pressures.

At a time when the midwifery profession, and the wider structure of maternity care, is a matter for popular and political debate, this book is a timely contribution. It will be an invaluable read for all those interested in maternity care in England.

Tania McIntosh is Lecturer in Midwifery at the University of Nottingham, UK. Initially trained as an historian, Dr McIntosh worked as a tutor in History at the University of Sheffield, until 2000 when she commenced midwifery training at the same university. Since then she has worked as a clinical midwife in Sheffield and at the City Hospital Nottingham. In 2009 she was one of the founders of De Partu, a national interdisciplinary research group for the history of midwifery and birth.

A Social History of Maternity and Childbirth

Key Themes in Maternity Care

Tania McIntosh

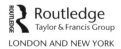

Routledge
Taylor & Francis Group

LONDON AND NEW YORK

RG
964
.G7
M35
2012

First published 2012
by Routledge
2 Park Square, Milton Park, Abingdon, Oxon, OX14 4RN

Simultaneously published in the USA and Canada
by Routledge
711 Third Avenue, New York, NY 10017

Routledge is an imprint of the Taylor & Francis Group, an informa business

British Library Cataloguing in Publication Data
A catalogue record for this book is available from the British Library

Library of Congress Cataloging in Publication Data
McIntosh, Tania.
A social history of maternity and childbirth : key themes in
maternity care / Tania McIntosh. -- 1st ed.
p. cm.
1. Maternal health services--Great Britain--History--20th century.
2. Childbirth--Great Britain--History--20th century. 3. Midwifery--Great
Britain--History--20th century. I. Title.
RG964.G7M35 2012
362.198'200941--dc23
2011038600

ISBN13: 978-0-415-56162-4 (hbk)
ISBN13: 978-0-415-56163-1 (pbk)
ISBN13: 978-0-203-12422-2 (ebk)

Typeset in Times
by Taylor & Francis Books

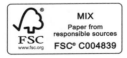

MIX
Paper from
responsible sources
FSC
www.fsc.org FSC® C004839

Printed and bound in Great Britain by
CPI Antony Rowe, Chippenham, Wiltshire

Contents

Tables

Preface

Any book written says as much about the author as it does about its subject, and this volume is a prime example. I came to the topic both as an historian and a midwife, in that order. In the early 1990s I took a degree in history, focusing on the social and economic history of early twentieth-century Britain, followed by a master's degree in English Local History and a dissertation that focused on the decline of Stourbridge Fair in Cambridge, originally one of the largest trading fairs in the country. However, my research world, together with my life, was turned upside down by my experience of the pregnancy and birth of my first child in 1992. Casting around for a PhD topic, I was drawn to the exploration of a profession and an experience that had never crossed my radar before, and I settled down to investigate the history of maternity care and midwifery in Sheffield between 1879 and 1939. During this time I had two further children of my own; the second born during the height of excitement around *Changing Childbirth*, and the third a planned home birth for which I had to argue (only with the doctors; the midwife was hugely supportive). My research was always an intersection between the personal and the intellectual; I remember sitting in the secretary's office at the Jessop Hospital in Sheffield trying to concentrate on nineteenth-century annual reports of the hospital and being distracted by my own baby kicking inside me. I obtained my PhD in the same year that my third child was born, and despite moving into history teaching at the University of Sheffield, found myself increasingly drawn to midwifery. Two things finally pushed me; not getting a Wellcome grant for which I had applied, and the midwife who had delivered my daughter saying to me, in relation to midwifery, 'If you don't try you'll never know.' So I tried, and spent three years training as a midwife, and a further four practising clinically, first in Sheffield and then in Nottingham. My 'day job' now is as a Lecturer in Midwifery, educating further generations of aspiring midwives and supporting them through academic and pastoral crises and being hugely proud of them in their successes. My research love has, however, remained history and in particular the history of maternity, and it is to this that I have returned whenever I have time.

One of the issues which I have always found interesting is that midwives are fascinated by the history of their profession, and historians have in turn, increasingly mined the history of maternity. Yet even with the move of midwifery education into the university sector in the 1990s, there has been very little cross-fertilisation between midwives and historians, despite the fact that midwives are increasingly undertaking research and research degrees in the area. It is perhaps a throwback to the days when medical men would write hagiographic memoirs of each other, and professional historians would disdain the work of 'amateurs'. Perhaps it is also a reflection of the lack of self-confidence that midwives have in their work, which means they do not submit papers for history conferences or journals. As an historian and a midwife I have tried to explore research and ideas from both traditions and to draw them together. I would hope that in the future, increasing use could be made by each group of the skills and insight of the other in order to develop a deeper and richer picture of one of the most fundamental of human experiences.

Acknowledgements

Thank you to:

Janette Allotey, Julia Allison, Mavis Kirkham, Billie Hunter and everyone on the Steering Group of *De Partu*; John Woodward; Seán Lang; Cate Hammond; Pam Hancock; Alice Bigelow; my colleagues in the Academic Division of Midwifery at the University of Nottingham, particularly Cathy Ashwin; Diane Fraser; my colleagues on Bonington Ward and Labour Suite at Nottingham City Hospital; Libby Milne; Dorothy Johnston and Caroline Kelly from The University of Nottingham Special Collections; Denise Amos; Sarah Badcock from the Department of History at the University of Nottingham; Lyn Balmforth at the NCT; Irene Boston for transcription; Jean Robinson, Sheila Kitzinger and Janet Balaskas for allowing me to interview them; all the retired midwives who allowed me to interview them; my students, particularly 0803 for being my 'first' group.

The University of Nottingham New Researchers Fund for a grant to pilot an oral history of midwifery.

My children: Owen, Seán and Caitlin.

My parents: André and Pam.

And especially Becky; and not just for dealing with the references ...

Abbreviations

AIMS	Association for Improvements in Maternity Services
ARM	Association of Radical Midwives
BMJ	*British Medical Journal*
CMB	Central Midwives Board
DHSS	Department of Health and Social Security
GP	general practitioner
LGB	Local Government Board
MMR	maternal mortality rate (deaths per thousand births)
MoH	Medical Officer of Health
NBTF	National Birthday Trust Fund
NCA	Natural Childbirth Association (later the NCT)
NCT	National Childbirth Trust
NHS	National Health Service
NMC	Nursing and Midwifery Council
NPEU	National Perinatal Epidemiology Unit
RCM	Royal College of Midwives
RCOG	Royal College of Obstetricians and Gynaecologists
UKCC	United Kingdom Central Council (for nursing, midwifery and health visiting)

Introduction

> Choices about birth are never as simple as selecting a can of beans from a supermarket shelf. They often involve powerful emotions – hope, fear, anger, guilt – to name a few. It is understandable that this should be so because birth is not just a matter of pushing a baby out of your body, a demonstration of bio-mechanics, but concerns fundamental human *values*.
>
> (Kitzinger 1988: 10)

Sheila Kitzinger, one of the most famous and influential voices in the story of maternity care in the twentieth century, wrote these words in 1988, a time when 99 per cent of births took place in some kind of institutional setting, usually an NHS hospital with full obstetric facilities. Regardless of the social class of the mother, the majority of babies were delivered by a midwife who was nearly always a woman, was also a qualified nurse and had undergone the majority of her training in an NHS hospital. In an emergency situation any senior doctor who attended a woman in labour would be a member of RCOG and would have chosen obstetrics and gynaecology as their speciality. During pregnancy and after the birth, women were seen by their GP and their community midwife, who was usually linked to several GP practices. If a woman was having her second or third baby, and had a blameless medical and obstetric history, then she may have been allowed to have a home birth in the attendance of a community midwife; only 0.9 per cent of women gave birth at home in 1988. As seen from Kitzinger's language, the concept of 'choice' was just beginning to develop in the maternity services, often driven by women themselves who were increasingly loath to accept the paternalism of the midwifery and obstetric professions when it came to making decisions about their pregnancy, their birth and their baby.

By 2002, ideas about 'choice' and 'control' in maternity were central to policies and protocols from ward level to national government. 'Women centred care', in which the care offered was based on rigorously assessed research evidence, was the only acceptable style of provision, with women and professionals expected to be equal partners in decision making. The reasons for this sea change are complex and their roots can be traced to broader social change in the period, including smaller family size and the feminist discourse. Underneath the language, however, hospital remained the most usual place of birth, with midwives still delivering the majority of babies but with Caesarean section accounting for around a quarter of all deliveries. The midwife working on the labour suite, on the wards or in the community would now be likely to have a diploma or degree in her subject and would have been educated within a university setting as much as in the hospital.

At the beginning of the period of this book a pregnant woman would have recognised very few of the features of maternity care that were mainstream by the late 1980s let alone the early twenty-first century. She too was most likely to be delivered by a midwife, but the birth would take place in the home, and in an emergency a GP would come to the house, providing that one could be found and there was money to pay the fee. The midwife herself was unlikely to be trained although she probably had many years of experience in her work, and she worked independently charging a few shillings for attendance at the birth. There were no choices to be made about antenatal or postnatal care, as neither of these things had been developed, although many midwives in poorer districts would come in for several days after the birth to cook and clean and attend to the baby. Completed family size was falling, although large families remained the norm in some communities, including those in coal-mining or steel-making areas. Death in childbirth was a risk, but infant death an even greater one, with around 150 babies per 1,000 dying before their first birthday in some areas.

Throughout the century the experience of maternity seemed never to be far from the minds not just of women having babies, or indeed of their doctors and midwives, but also of health officials, journalists, statisticians, sociologists and policy makers. It is a truism to say that pregnancy and birth are at the same time intensely private and uniquely public, but in this period they stepped out of the shadows and became central to social discourse as well as being influenced by it. This book focuses on some, but by no means all, of these threads because the centrality of birth to society and to life means that it is possible to trace its social history in many ways. This book is one of many which could be written and which would all tell the story in different ways, highlighting different developments and issues. Stories told around the history of birth have tended to be written in oppositional terms; doctors against midwives, professionals against consumers, men against women. These stories have been very influential in discussions of birth, highlighting both its importance and the different 'spin' which can be put on it to suit contemporary pre-occupations as much as historical enquiry. This book is equally partial in its approach, partly because the subject is vast, and partly because so many areas are, as yet, little explored. It seeks to show broadly how maternity care developed in England in the twentieth century, and to consider reasons for the biggest changes across the period. Underlining these developments is what might be termed the 'regulation of birth'. Too important to be left to chance, much less to untrained women, birth became codified in a variety of ways across the period; through the education and registration of midwives, the expression of ideas around 'risk', the development of official and technical surveillance of both mother and foetus, and society's growing involvement in every aspect of pregnancy and birth, from who should become a mother to what they should eat and where and how they should deliver. This book focuses on the regulation of birth, by individuals, consumer groups, professions and society. It also develops the idea, often forgotten in histories of maternity, that women, as mothers and as consumers of maternity care, were never passive vessels, but always had agency. They chose to accept or reject certain treatments or types of care, and for some women at some time, even relinquishing power could be a choice. The growing hospitalisation of birth across the twentieth century, for example, did not occur simply because women were forced into it by powerful doctors and passive midwives; it occurred at different rates in different areas for a variety of reasons which included social and economic factors as well as beliefs about the availability of particular interventions or techniques and ideas about risk and safety.

The book traces the intersection of mothers and their care givers, particularly midwives, and the ways in which their experience of maternity changed between 1902 and 2002. Using a variety of sources it tries to illuminate not just the dominant discourse at any one point, but also the stories which do not quite fit, such as the enthusiastic take up of technology by some midwives, or demands by women for hospital births rather than home births. Inevitably a book such as this relies very much on the work done by others. Histories of maternity have been told in broad-based terms, but particular aspects have also been considered using detailed archival work on issues such as maternal mortality or around specific localities. In writing this book a variety of sources have been used, both work done by many historians, and original primary sources. Of particular value have been the collections of letters and oral histories which tell mothers' stories in their own words; these include Llewelyn Davies' famous collection of *Letters From Working Women*, first published in 1915, as well as later compilations including oral histories by Smith and Devlin. There are, inevitability, a lot of issues not considered in this work, including infant feeding, the impact of immigration or older motherhood, the position of fathers, or the wider ramifications of the permissive society. This is not for lack of will; all or any of these topics would add depth and richness to the story, and hopefully someone will be inspired to tell these, and other, stories.

After several books on the history of midwifery were published in the 1980s and 1990s, the field has been relatively quiet, although papers and journal articles have continued to appear. There are signs, however, that maternity is once again being re-examined by historians with the recent book by Reid (2011) focusing on the history of midwifery in Scotland, and the forthcoming publication of a monograph by Davis on motherhood in the second half of the twentieth century, as well a comparative volume exploring the history of nursing and midwifery edited by Borsay and Hunter. Reid and Hunter are midwives first and foremost, Davis and Borsay are historians. Cross-disciplinary work, to which this book contributes in small measure, can give context to histories of maternity by allowing for different perspectives and different approaches. It is to be hoped that this book will be useful to historians, midwives and others exploring the history of maternity, and that its arguments and omissions will inspire further research in the area.

The book is divided into chronological chapters which roughly correspond to significant features in the history of maternity care in England. It begins in 1902 with the passing of the first English Midwifery Act, and ends with a new regulatory landscape for midwives and a conference exploring the apparently unstoppable rise of the Caesarean section. In-between it focuses on the development of midwifery and medicine in relation to maternity, and considers the role of women in the changing story of birth. Alongside these issues the book explores the influence of wider social concerns and pressures; pregnancy and birth never occurred in a vacuum in the twentieth century but were always part of wider debates about health, welfare, and the relationship between society and its citizens.

1 Historiography and comparisons

Introduction

Writing about the history of maternity and midwives has always been driven by complex contemporary agendas. This is apparent in not only the English but the international context, and has impacted also on sociological explorations of this most fundamental of human experiences. The stories of maternity have been written by doctors, and more recently by midwives, with themselves as centre stage. Sociologists and statisticians have mined the history of birth in support of arguments about the meaning of profession, the subjection of women, or of the misuse of power and technology in the name of safety. This chapter will explore some of these issues and the impact that they have had on thinking and writing about the history of maternity. History writing should, as far as is humanly possible, put the story in the context of its time and not judge it by contemporary mores or paradigms. This is never easy as the writer is the product of their times and carries beliefs and prejudices so ingrained as to be invisible. However, it is possible to explore not only the stories that have been written, but to consider what purpose they served.

The first section of this chapter will concentrate on the historiography of maternity, birth and midwifery. Much of the work that has been published is reductionist in nature, and has focused on the positives or negatives of progress. The language used is that of 'fights', 'battles' and 'campaigns' won and lost, whether for the regulation of midwifery, the provision of analgesia in labour, or beliefs about the relative safety of one birthing environment over another. In the late twentieth century, as women began to tell their stories, similar language was used. The story of maternity is therefore a maelstrom of military language, often told in oppositional terms. This appears paradoxical when pregnancy and birth are quintessentially about nurture and development.

However, over the last 20 years a different strand in writing has developed, which looks at specific issues often using very detailed archive work. The outstanding example of this is Loudon's book *Death in Childbirth* (1992) which explored the history of maternal mortality in twentieth-century Britain, and put it firmly in an international context. His work highlighted the multiplicity of factors at work in the maintenance of a relatively high level of maternal death rate, and in its final precipitous decline (in Western countries at least). This chapter will consider the ways in which this type of history has deepened and contextualised the stories told by great men and angry women, and how it carries its own ingrained truths and beliefs. Birth is publically mediated, but is also an intensely private and personal event. Historians have argued that the shift to hospital birth in particular exemplified the move of discourse around birth from the private domestic sphere to the institutional public one. Yet in all these debates the voice often lost is that of women who often did not leave written evidence of their beliefs and experiences. In order to capture these voices, this chapter will explore new approaches to what constitutes historical evidence and how it is gathered, in an effort to bring mothers back into the central drama of their own lives: pregnancy and birth.

The study of sociology has played a significant role in shaping the story of maternity. A large part of the writing on midwifery in particular is based around attempts to promote or destroy the concept of midwifery as a highly skilled occupation. Within this strand there has been much written about the relevance of the concept of profession to work such as midwifery, and whether it better conforms to subsets such as semi-profession, leaving the female midwife under the thumb of the obstetrician. All writing on midwifery history incorporates the idea of the profession and this has had a significant impact not only on attitudes to midwives and midwifery, but also the way maternity history is conceptualised.

Beyond issues of professional status, the way maternity is viewed by society has a huge impact not only on the way that the service has developed but also the kinds of stories which are told about it. Ideas of deference – women to men, everyone to the medical profession for example – have impacted on how and where birth is experienced. Waves of feminist thinking and action have also been central to readings of maternity. This might include women's demands for pain relief, for hospital births and home helps, as well the influential work of women like Sheila Kitzinger and Ann Oakley in Britain who helped to drive the demands of women to wrest control of their maternities back from the paternalistic experts. Debates around birth have never taken place in the sterile atmosphere of medical discourse; birth is so central to the way a society sees itself that discussion is always broad and often heated. Similarly, the history of maternity cannot be viewed in isolation, but must be seen as part of the history of the way society sees itself.

Although all of the above issues are pertinent to the English story, which is the one which this book will be telling, it is important to put maternity into its international context. Just as in Britain, it is the 'fight' for midwifery which has formed the central tier of writing about maternity in countries such as Canada, the USA, India and South Africa. This chapter will analyse the ways in which other countries tell their stories of maternity, and highlight the themes which other cultures see as central to the telling of birth.

This chapter will therefore place the history of maternity in twentieth-century England in a wider thematic and conceptual context.

Historiography of maternity

Much of the traditional writing on the history of maternity has come from the twin spectra of Whig history and what might be termed 'great men' (Versluysen 1980). The term 'Whig history' was coined in 1930s by historian Herbert Butterfield to describe the writing of history as that of the inexorable rise of enlightened progress; where every development leads to the sunlit perfection of today (Butterfield 1931). In a similar vein, there is the thesis that history is always written by the winners (Carr 1961), and this certainly appears to be true of a large proportion of the histories of maternity (Davies 1980: 11). The impression has always been given that maternity and care around childbirth particularly progressed and improved through the work of significant individuals. The story of the growing involvement of men in midwifery care during the seventeenth and eighteenth centuries is told as a series of names: Chamberlen, Smellie, Hunter (Radcliffe 1967). The Chamberlen family developed the midwifery forceps, and thereby transformed the safety of birth (Radcliffe 1947). The argument was that women previously left to die undelivered by midwives who just sat and watched, could now be saved by mechanical intervention. Smellie and Hunter not only lectured on midwifery, to both men and women, but also wrote about it, giving their philosophies and ideas a wider range and longer life span (Smellie 1752).

The medical profession has always been adept at celebrating those who came before them, and the stories of great men are often told by their successors. For an area such as midwifery this was particularly true as the nineteenth century saw the carving out of the specialised niche which would later call itself 'obstetrics' (Arney 1982; Drife 2002; Weisz 2005). It derived from 'man-midwifery', but saw itself as set apart in the sense that it was involved with delineating the normal as much as the pathological. That the speciality was a late developer and seen by more prestigious branches of medicine as lacking in complexity or taste, seems to have made obstetricians all the more determined to stake their claim. They were also wary of the charge of simply doing women's work, and much of the hagiographic writing on great obstetricians was written in order to highlight their uniquely positive, and male, contribution to the story of maternity (Radcliffe 1947; Munro Kerr et al. 1954; Radcliffe 1967; Willocks and Barr 2004).

Obscure biographies written by now obscure men may at first appear irrelevant to the wider story of maternity, but the arguments they used and the issues they highlighted have made an impact beyond their numbers. Alongside the battles between doctors and midwives for the control of childbirth in twentieth-century England, was an equally significant one fought between general practitioners (GPs) and obstetricians. This story is seldom told however because GPs lost. In the nineteenth century locally based doctors, who worked outside the big hospitals and complex hierarchies of medicine, were building their practices as 'family doctors' (Loudon 1984). They attended births and visited ailing children, they dealt with fevers, accidents, injuries, and chronic conditions. At the end they helped to safeguard a good death and wrote the death certificate. As part of the community, the literature suggested that they were highly valued and the concept of the family doctor is still held dear by many in England today. However, as far as the increasingly specialised hospital-based medical profession was concerned, GPs were the jack of all trades and the masters of none. Their skill around childbirth was particularly mocked, and the need for specialist obstetricians constantly debated (Loudon 2008). This has had an impact on the way that maternity care is organised even now.

It was not just 'great men' whose lives and works have been celebrated in the stories of maternity; there have been great women too. Some of the most famous of these, such as Jane Sharpe and Louise Bourgeois who worked in England and France respectively in the early modern period, have been written about extensively by those who wish to put midwives back into childbirth (Hobby 1999). In an opposite twist to Whig history, these women are often held up as a model to follow and seen as shining lights for the cause of midwifery and women after whom things started to go wrong. More broadly, historians have argued that midwives in early modern England were highly regarded within their communities (Harley 1993; Allison personal communication). However, even for those midwives who were Church licensed and pillars of their community, there has lingered the suspicion that they were potentially engaged in superstition, witchcraft, abortion and infanticide (Forbes 1962; Forbes 1966; Harley 1990; King 1993). The debate between historians who characterise midwives of the time as eminently respectable and knowledgeable and those who believe that they trod the wilder shores of practice has been highly polarised and has sometimes been weakened by a lack of appreciation about social concepts of health and illness, which were very different in the early modern period (Porter 1997). Concepts such as 'superstition' are slippery and value-driven and need to be seen in the context of their time; it may be that in future a late twentieth-century belief in the ability of technology to reduce the risks of birth may come to be characterised as 'superstition'. Nevertheless the power and influence of some midwives in the sixteenth and seventeenth centuries seems all the more remarkable in view of the decline in the status of midwifery which was perceived to follow (for one of the earliest readings of this in sociological terms, see Clark 1919: 242). However, after the supposed 'dark ages' of the eighteenth and nineteenth centuries in terms of midwifery, there has been a twentieth-century surge in 'great' women who have been involved in maternity. Some of these women, like Rosalind Paget who was a founder member of the Royal College of Midwives (RCM), were midwives (Hannam 1997). Many more however have been non-midwives, vocal in the late twentieth century for the way in which they have championed the cause of women; often the forgotten voice in maternity. Sheila Kitzinger, a redoubtable campaigner for women's rights around birth and sexuality was described by *The Guardian* newspaper on the dust-jacket of one of her books, as 'hav[ing] done for birth what Florence Nightingale did for nursing and

Marie Stopes did for contraception' (Kitzinger 2000). Similarly, the active birth campaigner Janet Balaskas is credited almost single-handedly with getting labouring women off beds and onto mats, bean bags and their feet (Kitzinger's foreword in Balaskas 1991). These women are not midwives but, like the great doctors before them, are charged with having not only changed the history of maternity, but improved it.

One strand of history writing in midwifery and maternity which has been particularly powerful is that of what might be termed conflict writing, whereby those with an axe to grind put down another group in a contemporary dispute under the aegis of historical writing. This writing has often been highly polemical. The trend started with doctors, anxious to carve out a respectable and lucrative corner of midwifery practice. James Aveling, a nineteenth-century doctor with ambition (he founded the Jessop Hospital for Women in Sheffield and the Chelsea Hospital for Women in London) was one of the earliest chroniclers of the history of midwifery (Aveling 1872). He had many irons in the fire, not least his scheme for the training and regulation of midwives as subordinates to doctors. He described midwives as dangerous and ignorant in their practice, and as responsible for high rates of maternal death. However, while many contemporaries used similar rhetoric as a reason to argue that midwifery should be outlawed, Aveling suggested that they could be rehabilitated under suitable medical supervision. His historical writing was therefore designed to support him in arguing his political point. All historical writing needs to be seen, as far as possible, in the context of the time in which it was written; it is never unbiased and never without a wider agenda. Maternity, wrapped as it is in social meaning, its rituals reflecting the concerns of society around it is particularly susceptible to contemporary readings. In the late nineteenth and early twentieth century the image of the dirty, ignorant, gin-swilling midwife, developed by writers such as Aveling, was shorthand for everything that was wrong in maternity care. Sarah Gamp, Dickens' portrayal of a nurse-midwife in *Martin Chuzzlewit*, as happy at a laying out as a lying in, was frequently pressed into service as an awful warning to those who would not accept progress (Bullough 1917; Summers 1989).

Conflict writing has remained a powerful tradition in histories of English maternity, but has increasingly been written by women from a feminist perspective. One of the most notable proponents of this style of writing has been Donnison, who wrote a powerful and detailed account focusing on the battle for the legal foundation of midwifery and whose book is still the touchstone for those referencing the history of the maternity services (Donnison 1988). It put the story of registration and its aftermath in the social context of the battle between midwives and doctors for 'the control of childbirth' as it was described in the subtitle. This perspective was partly influenced by the time in which Donnison wrote; the 1970s and 1980s saw the development of a rhetoric of birth based on feminism, the language of disempowerment, and the demand for re-empowerment. In representing this 'struggle' as a linear one between two occupational groups scrapping for professional hegemony,

Donnison marginalised the role of women as service users in shaping their own reproductive destinies and this is an omission that has been perpetuated by other histories (Oakley 1984; Towler and Bramall 1986). Donnison's work has continued to exert a powerful influence over the way that the story of maternity has been told. But the sense of maternity as a battleground has been evinced in other areas. Heagerty (1996) wrote of the conflict between elite educated midwives and untrained midwives. In her reading, trained midwives, represented by Paget and the College of Midwives, sought to marginalise the work of midwives who continued to give care in the traditions of pre-registration times. Heagerty described statutory supervision of midwives in particular as a powerful tool of social control, used not only by doctors against midwives, but by midwives to discredit their rivals. Midwifery writers such as Kirkham (1996) have drawn on this reading to inform their own work on contemporary supervision, although Hannam (1997) argued that Heagerty's reading was too simplistic and that early midwifery leaders had considerable sympathy with, if not always a thorough understanding of, the plight of working-class midwives.

The sense of conflict and the idea of maternity as a battleground developed between doctors and midwives, but in the atmosphere of the 1970s and 1980s an equally powerful debate emerged with motherhood at its heart. This was in many ways a pivotal moment because although the voices of women had been heard, off camera as it were, through the medium of social surveys and enquiries (Llewelyn Davies 1915; Spring Rice 1939; RCOG 1948) this was the first time that women began to develop their own rhetoric around the meaning and practice of maternity. One of the greatest exponents of polemical writing with mothers at its heart has been Kitzinger, who wrote *The Experience of Childbirth* in 1962 and has continued to develop her philosophy into the new millennium (see bibliography for details of her main works). In her writing, and in the work of Balaskas (1991, 1992), there was a new battleground; that between women and everything that represented control and power, whether it was doctors or midwives, machinery or protocols (Kitzinger 2002). For women to have the experience they wanted was seen as a fight in which allies and weapons were required (Thomas 1996). The way in which the story of the history of maternity is told – with midwives forced into subjugation by doctors, or women forced to give birth in hospital rather than at home – is relevant not only to historians but to all who are involved in maternity today. The rhetoric of conflict and control continues to exert a powerful influence on the way in which maternity is viewed and experienced.

Beyond the broad-brush approach to maternity history, which has concentrated on concepts of professional takeover and loss and on issues of power and control, there is another strand in the historiography of the subject which focuses on the detail of particular areas. Within her writing Donnison exemplified this approach with her detailed examination of the development of midwifery registration in the late nineteenth century. Another hugely influential writer has been Irvine Loudon, a retired GP turned medical historian, whose work on maternal mortality suggested that traditional midwives offered far safer care than their medical rivals, and whose work has been referenced by policy makers as much as historians (Berridge 2005, 2008). Other writers have built on his work to develop an increasingly nuanced picture of maternity history, based primarily on detailed local or regional studies of care, including work by Marks on East London (1994, 1995, 1996), Peretz on Oxfordshire (1990, 1992) and McIntosh on Sheffield (1997, 1998, 2000). Although most of these have remained in the domain of historians, and have been published in historical collections and journals, some studies have had a wider impact. In particular, Allison's work (1996), which was a painstaking exploration of the work of district midwives in Nottingham between 1948 and 1974, has proved central to contemporary debates about the work of midwives (Report of the Expert Maternity Services Group 1993; Allison 1994). Her research included oral interviews with several retired midwives, and the evidence she obtained was woven in with the evidence from the birth registers they had kept as well as official records such as Medical Officer of Health reports. The use of primary evidence such as this is fraught with logistical difficulties; not least because in England the survival of records is so patchy (Nicol and Sheppard 1985; McGann 1997; Allotey and McIntosh 2009). Hospitals are under an obligation to retain maternity records for 25 years in case of litigation, but thereafter most records are destroyed because there is no space to save them long term. District midwives, who undertook the bulk of maternity care in England until the 1974 reorganisation of the maternity services, kept registers of all their cases, together with records of their controlled drugs. Again survival depends on the individual; the records are highly personal, recording details of names, addresses and ages of mothers as well as details of their labour and puerperium. The legitimacy or otherwise of the baby is recorded together with any remarks when the baby was born or died under suspicious circumstances. Often the families of retired midwives have destroyed case registers after the death of the midwife because of the sensitivity of the information contained within them. There is as yet in England no preservation policy for such records. In fact the hundred year rule which already exists and is used to protect sensitive information contained in census records for example can equally be applied to midwifery records; which can be an unrivalled source of evidence for everything from midwifery workloads, to obstetric interventions and rates of breastfeeding (McIntosh 2010, 2011).

Allison's book used another source of evidence which is increasingly being explored in order to elucidate the experiences and beliefs of those who would otherwise leave no written record. She used oral interviews to explore in detail the work of the district midwives whom she studied. Oral history developed credence in the 1960s in particular with the development of the writing of history from below, and has been used effectively to study marginalised groups (Perks and Thomson 1998). It has also been used to explore a wide range of health issues, exemplified by Bornat's edited volume which considered subjects such as learning disability, abuse in healthcare settings, and HIV/

AIDS as well as more mainstream topics like midwifery (Bornat et al. 1999). As many commentators have observed, the construction of oral history has its pitfalls, particularly around the issues of selective memory and respondents telling the stories or giving the opinion that they think the interviewer wants to hear. Oakley, writing from a sociological point of view, has written of the effect of the unequal power relationship between interviewer and interviewee and the impact that this can have (1981). Yow (2006) explored the subjectivity of the relationship between interviewer and interviewee, arguing that although this made historians wary of using the methodology, a growing appreciation of reflexivity within oral history has allowed researchers to acknowledge and even to appreciate the nuances of subjective storytelling. Clearly there is always the risk that the interviewer does not hear what they want or expect to hear. A good example of this is *The Midwife's Tale* by Leap and Hunter (1993); another book which has continued to be highly influential. The authors were both midwives, and were seeking evidence for the 'golden age' of midwifery, when midwives were independent, autonomous and skilled in the art of midwifery rather than the science of obstetrics. What they in fact found after a series of interviews with midwives who had worked in the 1920s and 1930s, including one untrained handywoman, was that the midwives did not appear to possess many of the qualities or skills which the authors were expecting to find. Equally thought-provoking, argued, was the fact that the handywoman they interviewed was not a caring repository of traditional knowledge but appeared to be quite the opposite.

The idea of using oral interviews to explore the experiences of women, rather than of midwives, was used initially in the social sciences; the work of Oakley (1981) being particularly important. Her research on the experience of pregnancy and motherhood undertaken in the mid-1970s is now equally powerful as historical evidence around maternity care in that period. However, apart from the work of Allison and Leap and Hunter, historians are only just beginning to explore the use of oral history to study maternity and women's sexuality (Davis 2011; Fisher 2008; Szreter and Fisher 2010; Reid 2011) although there is a published strand of storytelling which is a powerful, if sometimes unfocused way of bringing the past to life (Aspinall et al. 1997; Smith 1997; Worth 2007). Verbal rather than written storytelling has a long tradition in maternity (Kirkham and Perkins 1997). It ranges from the 'old wives' tales' that midwives and doctors warn their patients against (Bourne 1989), to the shared experiences discussed between new mothers, and the memories that midwives share on long night shifts. It is a way of passing on not only knowledge, but belief systems, and although hidden to formal written histories, it is an important component of the way mothers and midwives see each other and those who came before them. New technology is beginning to allow for the democratisation of history, particularly through the use of storytelling (see for example www.nursevoices.org.uk, an oral history of nursing, and www.healthtalkonline.org, which is not strictly history but uses interviewing to allow recipients of care to tell their stories). It has the potential to allow a multiplicity of voices to be heard and recognised, although its use is still in its infancy and remains to be fully explored.

This brief delve into the historiography of writing on maternity demonstrates in microcosm the way in which history develops. In the wider historical context there is a contemporary move away from Whig or anti-Whig history, and a resurgence of narrative history. Davies (1980: 12) argued that narrative history lacks 'comparison, criticism and reflection' and it certainly implies that the story will have a beginning, a middle and an end, although in reality history is messy, full of switchbacks and blind alleys. Sometimes, however, it may be the seemingly insignificant moments which illuminate the landscape most clearly and can be missed if theory building is foregrounded (Carr 1961).

The sociological context of maternity history

The experience of maternity, whether as a mother or as a care giver, has never existed in a social vacuum. There are biological elements of the experience which are unchanging, although it has been argued that even these can vary so significantly in interpretation as to seem like a different phenomenon (Hobby 1999; Allotey 2007), but pregnancy and birth are fundamental to how a society sees itself. As such they are hedged around with ritual and superstitions, whether to ward off the threat of death or to celebrate the arrival of the next generation and the continuum which that implies. It is through the lens of ritual and belief that society makes sense of birth, and of the strength and vulnerability of its women at this time.

Ideas of ritual and belief suggest primitive birth cultures, where women birth surrounded by other women and safe from the demands of time limits and technology. This idea has exerted a powerful fascination with Western cultures particularly in the second half of the twentieth century, where 'primitive' as applied to birth ceased to be pejorative and became something to be celebrated (Kitzinger 2000; Priya 1992; Walsh 2007). The pictures and stories were of strong women, comfortable in their own bodies and free from the dictates of doctors, policies and their own fears. The same reading was used earlier in the twentieth century to draw distinctions between the perceived needs of middle- and upper-class women and their working-class sisters (Leavitt 1986). Working-class women were held to carry their pregnancies more easily and to birth with minimal assistance, simply because they were not refined. They had held onto their primitive instincts, whereas better-off women, not used to manual labour, found pregnancy a difficult and dangerous business. Grantly Dick-Read, the American pioneer of 'natural childbirth', theories around which he developed in the 1930s, drew on beliefs around primitive and working-class cultures to develop his ideas. He argued in successive articles and books that he had witnessed women in Africa giving birth without apparent pain, and a young working-class woman in the USA doing the same thing (Dick-Read 1933, 1942). His theories around the fear–tension–pain triad in labour drew on these experiences and were aimed at, and most enthusiastically taken up by, middle-class women (The National Childbirth Trust were initially Dick-Read proselytisers).

The concept of 'good' or 'bad' births has been a powerful one in stories of maternity, with the frames of reference changing over time. At various times, by various groups in society, different types of birth attendant and different types of ritual have been considered 'good' or 'bad'. In the 1920s for example it was considered by obstetricians to be bad to have to labour at home with only the local midwife for company, in the sense that it was potentially dangerous. By the end of the century, this situation was considered to be the apogee of a good birth (Cairns 2006). In the 1930s, midwives prided themselves on delivering babies over an intact perineum. This was partly a reflection of what they saw as their skill, and partly a commentary on the fact that midwives did not suture, so a doctor would have to be called out, with all the ritual and expense which that entailed for the mother. Conversely, by 1978 a 'good' birth, in obstetric terms, included an episiotomy in 53 per cent of cases; designed to protect the baby's head and to provide a cleaner, 'safer' wound than a natural tear would leave (Graham 1997; Macfarlane et al. 2000). In the early twenty-first century, episiotomy has again fallen out of favour and an intact perineum is to be prized, with a tear as second best.

The concept of 'good' and 'bad' has throughout history applied not only to the rituals of birth, but to mothers themselves. Different types of mother, and different types of mothering have been considered problematic and in need of regulation, depending on the wider preoccupations of society. One of the reasons for the introduction of the 1902 Midwives Act, and the maternal and infant welfare movement of which it was a part, was to address national concerns of 'deterioration'. At a time when Germany was militarising, and Britain had struggled to maintain its grip on South Africa during the Boer War, there was a sense that the nation itself had become innervated. One of the ways to address this was to be the glorification of the idea of motherhood, and exhortations to mothers to bring their children up to be worthy heirs of the Empire. Imperialist fear and ambition therefore found its way into bonny baby competitions, mothercraft classes, adverts for baby clothes and the work of midwives and sanitary inspectors (the forerunners of health visitors). Good mothers did not work outside the home or bottle feed their babies. Good mothers attended mothercraft classes given by experts so they knew best how to feed, clothe and rear 'king baby' as he (it was always a he) was known. Bad mothers were feckless and ignorant, a danger not only to themselves and their family but to the race as a whole (McIntosh 1997).

The rhetoric changed as the century developed but many of the same preoccupations lingered. Society no longer talks of race or Empire, but mothers who smoke, drink and bottle feed are considered beyond the pale and in need of 'education' and 'information'. Older mothers, once considered to be selfishly putting their own and their babies' lives in danger, are now considered to be acceptable, and even wise. Teenage mothers, with the connotations they carry of underage sex, of immaturity and irresponsibility are now helped to ensure that their mistake in getting pregnant does not ruin their lives and they do not do it again. Special classes and groups for pregnant teenagers, or drug users suggests goodwill and acceptance by society, but attendance and acceptance is bound up in a paternalistic and powerful view of what society actually wants from its parturient members (Apple 1995). The details have changed over time but history demonstrates that individuals have always operated within the belief systems of wider society; particularly with regard to something as fundamental as reproduction.

The economic and social trajectory of the century made an impact on the history of maternity; wealth and poverty both in terms of individuals and of society was significant, as were wider social preoccupations. Britain fought two major wars during this period, which were significant not only for the immediate impact they had on the lives of women, but on thinking about society in its broadest terms. During both the First and Second World Wars many women were employed outside the home for the first time (Thom 1998). Others, who had struggled through the Depression to keep their families afloat, now found they were richer than ever before with themselves working and their husbands receiving regular army pay. Average fertility rates dropped across the century, in all classes, and the growing rarity value of pregnancy potentially heightened awareness of it as a special time, and fuelled the need for it to be fulfilling and joyful (Hicks and Allen 1999; Macfarlane et al. 2000). Medical advances, spurred by the demands of war, in both the use of blood transfusion and antibiotics had a dramatic and lasting impact on maternal mortality (Loudon 1992). The welfare state and the National Health Service (NHS) were planned at the height of war (Webster 2002), and their impact on not only mothers, but on midwives and doctors was immediate and long lasting. Some historians have argued that war in the twentieth century has, apparently paradoxically, been a positive driver of change for women and children, due perhaps to an innate need to plan for a better future, of which maternity and children are the most potent symbols (Dwork 1987).

One area of social debate which has had a significant impact on the history of maternity is that of feminism; an area which this chapter has already touched on. The feminist debate which developed in the 1960s and 1970s had at its heart issues of empowerment and control, in areas as apparently diverse as the workplace and the bedroom. Superficially much of what was written and debated was extremely hostile to motherhood and to the nuclear family in particular (see for example Greer 1971). To be on equal terms with men meant to be without children; pregnancy, birth and motherhood tied women into a state of subjection. Underneath the rhetoric, however, the language and the concepts explored by feminists were vital in giving not only mothers but some midwives a new voice. Celebration of the power of the female body meant also the celebration of her ability to carry and birth a child (Phillips and Rakusen 1978; Kitzinger 2000). However, alongside the exploration of sexuality was the articulation of repression and regulation; in the case of mothers by the medical profession and their perceived handmaidens, midwives. Some women took the language of power and control and applied it to particularly the birthing experience; they argued for the right to informed consent for procedures, to deliver where and how they chose, and to make the systems-driven NHS more responsive to individual need. These debates impacted also on midwives and some, as women and as feminists, became involved in new midwifery groups such as Association of Radical Midwives (ARM). This group in particular supported the demands of women, but also made demands on the account of midwives themselves to be heard in a health service which increasingly seemed to marginalise their role.

However, even in the early twentieth century, the issues of women's rights and control over their bodies and health had at times been equally explicit, but are often lost to the sight of modern historians, because few ordinary women left any record of what they thought or felt about their lives. Contemporary groups such as the Women's Co-operative Movement strove to highlight the conditions in which women lived and raised families, and to call for state aid through the family allowance to go directly to mothers rather than through the male head of the family. Women such as Marie Stopes (Stopes 1919; Hall 2011) and Stella Browne (Browne et al. 1935; Hall 1997) campaigned for women to have control over their bodies in the areas of birth control and abortion. Beyond the headlines, in the day-to-day world of lives not recorded, women had abortions, demanded hospital birth and analgesia, demanded home birth in the face of obstetric disapproval, got up and did housework when they were ordered to stay in bed; private acts of feminism and female power (RCOG 1948; Szreter and Fisher 2010).

One of the over-arching themes of the twentieth century in all areas of society was industrialisation. School history taught that the industrial revolution occurred in the late eighteenth and early nineteenth centuries but in many ways it was the twentieth century that saw its full expression. This was particularly true for example of war, dehumanised and mechanised on a huge scale. In contrast pregnancy and birth were traditionally a quintessentially low-technology domestic experience. Yet in considering the trajectory of care in the twentieth century childbirth can be described as becoming 'industrialised', meaning the large-scale deployment of technology in the shape of monitors, scans, inductions and obstetric surgery. A lot of this was driven by concepts of 'safety' which became increasingly central to the discourse around maternity (Butler and Bonham 1963; Tew 1995). One of the most pervasive aspects of industrialisation is, however, that of time. The control of workers' lives through the use of time, and the ways in which they circumvented this in the nineteenth century was described by the historian E. P. Thompson (1967). Clock time, which in the pre-industrial era had not been the driving force in people's lives, now became pre-eminent. This preoccupation with time accelerated in the twentieth century and has become one of the main drivers in the delivery of maternity care, allied to the primacy of safety. Scans are used to pinpoint the day of delivery, and inductions of labour ordered if the pregnancy goes on too long. Partograms are used to delineate progress in labour, with action lines to prompt intervention if things are not happening at the obstetrically defined rate (see Chapter 5 for the developments of these technologies and their impact). For most of the period babies were limited in how much time they should spend at the breast, and wheels demonstrated baby's day parcelled into neat segments of sleep, feeding and play with the emphasis on clock-driven routine (Hardyment 2007).

The industrialisation of maternity has affected not only mothers and their babies, but their care givers. Until the mid-twentieth century most relationships between mothers and midwives were individual ones, negotiated on a personal basis. With the rise of the hospital as the default environment in which to birth, and the changing organisation of midwifery, the relationship became more impersonal and distant, and it became subject to greater regulation. The move of midwives from craftswomen to industrial workers has been seen by many as signalling the development of midwifery as a profession, with its own rules, training and regulation (McIntosh 1998; Dale and Fisher 2009). However, one of the main strands of historical debate around midwifery is the extent to which it has developed into a fully fledged profession. This has a contemporary impact, because midwives are encouraged to see themselves as professionals with the skills and knowledge to act autonomously. Historians of midwifery have dated the growing self-awareness of midwives to the time around the first English Midwives Act of 1902 (see Reid 2011 for parallel developments in Scotland). However, in the late twentieth century this belief clashed increasingly with the demands of time-driven maternity care, the dictates of state and hospital policies and the demands of women as consumers (Curtis et al. 2006). It nevertheless remains a central strand of how midwives see themselves, and its emergence as a concept deserves examination.

There has been a huge volume of work done by sociologists in particular on the development and hallmarks of professions. It has been argued that a profession can largely be defined by the control it exerts over its own entry, training, work, as well as in the alliances it makes with the State and other powerful organisations (Johnson 1972; although see Dent and Whitehead 2003 on recent changes to this hegemony). Medicine provides a powerful exemplar of this process (Larson 1977). Until the early nineteenth century it was largely unregulated, and though medical schools existed, the work was open to all comers (Smellie had no formal qualifications). The development of medicine as a closed profession occurred through a multiplicity of factors. Training schools developed, with systems of certificates and different levels of accreditation. Scientific and surgical advances meant that medicine was able to develop its own language and expertise and to control access to this through medical schools. The containment of the number of doctors being trained meant that, economically speaking, they had a scarcity value. This meant that they could charge for their time and expertise. The knowledge they carried also had a scarcity value; it was secret and not readily accessible to lay members of society. Finally, in order to develop an effective hegemony of practice a profession needs to be able to exert pressure through the apparatus of the State.

Again there is ample evidence throughout the nineteenth century of doctors doing this. A good example is their attitude to midwives, and their attempts to discredit their rivals by decrying their expertise. Aveling (1872) wrote of the dangers to society of untrained, ignorant and dirty midwives. By emphasising the effect on society as a whole, doctors such as Aveling were able to link their values to that of the State; they effectively promised to provide a more cost-effective service than midwives, in terms of lives saved and healthy populations ensured. Finally, again through the aegis of the State, medicine as a profession has managed to develop and retain its own system of regulation. It acts as its own gate-keeper not only in matters of entry to the profession, but also of exit in matters of dispute. It decides who practises, and disciplines those who it feels have overstepped the tenets of the profession (see Chapter 6 for the example of Wendy Savage). However, the majority of individual doctors, seeking to carve out a role for themselves through the development of a new speciality or technique, probably would not have viewed their position as part of an over-arching professional project. For most it was about individual livelihoods, and an often overpowering belief that what they were doing was for the good of society, however paternalistic that may have been.

Where then did this leave midwifery, a craft which had enjoyed at least equal status with surgeons and physicians in the pre-industrial era? Midwifery, together with nursing has been characterised by sociologists as a 'semi-profession' in the service of the male-dominated 'true' profession of medicine; specifically in this case of obstetrics (Etzioni 1969; Robinson 1990; Witz 1992). Many midwives would argue that midwifery has a lot of the hallmarks and demands of a true profession. To a certain extent the debate is one of semantics, but because of the impact that it has on how midwives see themselves, and society sees midwives, it is worth rehearsing. Midwives achieved a semi-closed shop with the passing of the first English Midwives Act in 1902, and this was strengthened with subsequent acts and rules which laid down entry gates, training periods, and the body of knowledge which a midwife was expected to possess. However, midwives have always worked with doctors, and the extent to which this has been a partnership or subordinate role has varied across the period on an organisational as well as on an individual level. Heagerty (1996) argued that the system of supervision set up at the time of the 1902 Act handed control of midwifery to a usually medical elite and was used to control every aspect of midwives' lives and work. Midwives who were quintessentially lower class were argued to be particularly victimised by the supervisory structure. Additionally, because midwives have, until the last decades of the twentieth century, been women, and medical hegemony was argued to be based on gender as well as class, it has been argued that they were at an additional disadvantage in pursuing a professional project in the face of a largely male medical profession (Cahill 2001). Instead Cahill, following the trajectory set by Donnison (1988), argued that male professional dominance through medicine led to a complete recasting of pregnancy and birth as a clinical and pathological process rather than a domestic and physiological one.

Towards the end of the twentieth century, with the emergence of a new feminist discourse, there has been an attempt to reinvigorate and to celebrate midwifery as a craft rather than as a profession (Gaskin 1975; ARM 1985); with the concept of 'profession' seen to have negative connotations of competition and exclusive expertise when women should be helping women. However, the rhetoric of profession has continued to exercise not only midwives but doctors as well and has shaped a lot of the discourse of maternity in the twentieth century. Most recently there has been debate around how far groups such as doctors and midwives retain their status as professionals given the rise of a management-led culture within the NHS (Carpenter 1977; Dent and Whitehead 2003). Equally pertinent to maternity care, as this book will explore, has been the perceived rise of 'patient power', partly as a result of pressure by consumer groups, but also as a result of the democratisation of medical information through the Internet and other electronic resources (Coulter 2002; see also Fannin 2006, for the use of the Internet for information sharing by midwives).

The international context

In the twentieth century midwifery was debated, regulated and even outlawed in various countries across the world. Many states became involved in prescribing ideal family size, and in policing motherhood through a network of public health initiatives, sanctions and even rewards. Different countries pursued different agendas depending on how midwives already worked, and what the medical profession and society saw as their role. Debates which left midwifery virtually destroyed in some American states, conversely led to midwives assuming a central role in reproductive health in the Netherlands. By the beginning of the new millennium the USA had an average Caesarean section rate of around 30 per cent compared to less than 15 per cent in the Netherlands, with the latter maintaining a home birth rate of 35 per cent; these two countries represent some of the extremes of the pathways followed by maternity services across the globe.

Writing on maternity from an international perspective demonstrates many of the same preoccupations with professionalism of midwifery, place of birth and the hegemony of technology that are seen in work on the English experience. Frequently the progress and outcome of regulation in England was the yardstick by which authors measured the achievements of other countries (Bourgeault 2006).

The contributors to Marland and Rafferty's (1997) exploration of maternity care in twentieth-century Europe explored the different agendas which prevailed in different countries. For the Netherlands there was a significant divide between trained and untrained midwives, both in terms of how they saw themselves and how they were seen by society (Marland 1997). Trained midwives were co-opted by the state to promulgate the public health agenda around issues of infant feeding, household hygiene and wider concepts of morality. In Denmark, by contrast, the agent for change was less about public health and more focused on private health with the emphasis on asepsis in midwifery care and personal cleanliness (Løkke 1997). Again, midwives were viewed as proselytisers for progress. As with English history, micro-studies have put flesh on the bones of wider ideas about how maternity fitted into a modern technologically mediated society.

Thompson (1997) wrote about the inception of the International Midwives Union (IMU; later became the International Confederation of Midwives, which still exists), a pan-European organisation founded in 1919. Just before the Second World War the IMU, which had representatives from 20 member countries, discussed the problems of competition from doctors and other health workers, the increased use of hospitals for delivery and the impact of the prolonged economic depression. The issue of other health workers encroaching on what the midwives saw as their occupational territory was a significant concern in the 1920s and 1930s. Nursing as a distinct occupation was developing as a result of its own regulation in many European countries. Whilst midwifery had always been recognised as a specialised role, nursing was much more fluid in its scope and as regulation began to occur so did the desire to carve out specific areas of occupational expertise (Fealy 2005). The growing band of district health visitors and nurses in particular were felt by midwives to impinge on their sphere of practice. They responded by actively engaging in a public health role, particularly around postnatal care (Sweet and Dougall 2008). This was an area in which midwives had previously had little involvement, and for nurses it was a good entry point into family work; in the USA in particular it was to give nurses significant leverage over the provision of wider maternity care. The division, or synthesis, between nursing and midwifery and the areas where nursing managed to stifle a separate midwifery profession have been particularly explored in relation to Canada where midwifery began to re-emerge in the early 1990s (Burtch 1994; Bourgeault 2006).

The birth rate fell dramatically across the century in most of the Western world, with expectations around the end of both World Wars. Causes and consequences have been much debated by historians, but not in relation to midwives whose livelihoods were on the line if numbers of babies being born declined dramatically. Fertility rates across Europe had varied with class throughout the nineteenth century; working-class couples tended to have larger families, for a variety of economic and social reasons. However, after a brief flurry at the end of the First World War, the birth rate nose-dived across most of the continent and there was much concerned talk of mothers 'striking' and of the increasing resort to birth control and abortion. As Thompson (1997) demonstrated, at least for the midwifery elite who attended the IMU, the situation left them in an awkward position. They had prided themselves on supporting women but with their livelihoods at stake, tension developed between what midwives saw as 'best' and what women wanted. Many governments developed pro-natalist policies in response to concerns about falling birth rates, particularly in a time of increased national tension in the 1930s when another major war was seen as increasingly likely. Governments in Germany and France, for example, struck medals which were given to women with larger families; women who were perceived to have done their duty to their nation as their men folk were expected to do on the battlefield. At the level of international debate midwives increasingly allied themselves with this pro-natalist movement. This left them following a paternalistic, and male-driven, agenda at the expense of the women they were supposed to be caring for. However, working in independent practice as most midwives did meant that they were paid by the case, and with increasing competition for work from doctors, nurses and institutions, midwives may have felt they had no choice but to support calls for a higher birth rate.

In many ways, European midwives were at liberty to debate these issues because although they saw their survival as being at stake, they were supported by regulation which defined their existence, even if it did not guarantee them work. The situation in the USA and Canada was very different, because the same conditions which had led to midwifery regulation in Britain and Europe led to emasculation in the New World. The debate had initially been conducted along similar lines to that in Europe with evidence of the increasing demonisation and marginalisation of traditional midwives. When midwifery did re-emerge in the USA, however, it was in the guise of the nurse-midwife who was overtly the handmaiden of obstetric science. Ladd-Taylor (1988) detailed the midwifery training required after the passing of the 1921 Sheppard-Towner Maternity and Infancy Protection Act, although she argued that concepts of professionalism (or semi-professionalism) did not reach into the remote South. The Act, although intended to safeguard midwives, helped to reduce their numbers by demanding a certain level of education; a double bind that was caused by attempts to 'professionalise' in several countries.

Despite this, even in North America the progression from 'social' to 'medical' discourses around childbirth was not linear. Doctors and midwives often worked in tandem, and used custom and ritual without a sense of opposition. Leavitt and Walton (1984) argued that in the USA, the fear of pain and debility, if not death, were important in shaping demands by women for different types of care. Dye (1986–87), who studied domiciliary care in New York in the early twentieth century, commented that 'poor and working class women were central to the transformation of birth from a social to a medical phenomenon.' She suggested that there was a struggle for power between doctors and patients as much as between doctors and midwives. Patients attempted to assert control by engaging a particular doctor or midwife, by resisting certain procedures (such as internal examinations) and by demanding others (especially analgesics). At the same time, doctors were trying to stamp their own authority on the situation by refusing to work in tandem with midwives, demanding the right to define active labour regardless of how the patient saw her progress, and by insisting on frequent internal examinations. Dye concluded that doctors were successful in medicalising childbirth before the rise of the hospital as the default place of delivery. Borst (1988), in her study of Wisconsin, noted the takeover of normal birth by family doctors, but found that midwives continued to operate in local communities along ethnic lines, and that their work combined elements of 'old' and 'new' craft. Women accepted doctors' views and expertise because they believed a safer and more scientific approach to birth was being offered and because doctors were respected members of the community in a way that midwives could not match. The choice was perhaps spurious because, as Borst noted, medical education was so sparse that doctors were unlikely to be better informed about birth than midwives. Women were nevertheless making their own decisions about the type of care they wanted, and the treatment they expected.

Writing on midwifery and birth in North America has developed alongside feminist scholarship from the 1970s onwards, and in tandem with the resurgence of the midwife. Direct entry training for midwives was recommended in Canada in the 1980s, following study of European models (Bourgeault et al. 2004). Tensions remained, however, between educated 'professionalised' midwives and 'craft' midwives in the USA. This included strong cultural and racial elements, with black and European immigrants seen as engaging in dangerous and unscientific practices (Hine 2005), rhetoric also heard in British debates about health in the colonies. Writing of India, for example, Lang (2007) identified multiple layers of beliefs operating in attempts to reduce maternal mortality, ranging from stereotypical ideas about the *dai* (traditional birth attendant) to concepts of the spread and defence of Empire. Thomas (2003) explored many of the same themes in her study of maternity in Kenya. More recently, Traditional Birth Attendants (TBAs) have been described by the World Health Organization as providing a bridge between old practices and new obstetrics, and as a result of this their work has been studied in a variety of historical contexts and locales. De Brouwere et al. (2002) took this one step further by using an historical analysis of maternal mortality in the Western world in the early twentieth century, and considering to what extent the trajectory of intervention could be traced in Third-World areas where death in childbirth remains a significant risk for mother and baby.

Conclusion

This chapter has briefly explored the historiography of maternity history, and has tried to place some of the themes of this book in a broader context. The main areas for enquiry by researchers have always been professionalisation of midwifery, the place of birth, and the recasting of maternity as a medical rather than social phenomenon. The history of midwifery has been seen by historians as a metaphor, or 'moral fable' for wider issues of health, control, gender and power. These factors are significant in the history of maternity, not only as they affected midwives, but for the impact they had on the experience of pregnant and birthing women. The development of a feminist rhetoric around maternity, which was taken up by midwives and women, had a significant effect on discourse from the 1970s to the present, and in turn had an impact on how history was seen and written. The history of maternity as written by doctors (and often promulgated by midwives; see Myles' midwifery textbooks) was seen as the march to enlightenment, with dirty domestic midwifery being displaced by clean, research-driven regulated care that had safety at its heart. This discourse continues to have a significant impact, but has been joined by the counter-argument that seeks to demonstrate the retreat from a golden age of domestic midwifery into industrial, impersonal modernity.

This book will explore these arguments and put them in their historical context. It will, however, also explore issues not covered in many traditional histories of midwifery and maternity, which have been touched on by this chapter. These range from deeply personal stories about what it was like to be a midwife or to have a baby at different points in the twentieth century to wider issues of the economic and social climate and the development of different models of health care. Maternity is intensely personal and at the same time uniquely public; it is driven by private desires and social discourses. This book will put these diverse drivers into their historical context in telling the story of maternity in twentieth-century England, and in exploring the variety of mechanisms by which it became proscribed and regulated.

2   1902–14

Introduction

In 1902, after many years of campaign and debate, the first English Midwives Act was passed. Midwives and historians have characteristically dated the growing self-awareness of midwives to this period, as a result of the provisions of the Act (Towler and Bramall 1986; Donnison 1988; Heagerty 1990; Fox 1993; Leap and Hunter 1993). The Act laid down rules about the training, registration and regulation of midwives as well as a timetable for the gradual elimination of the untrained midwife. The background to the passing of the Act, together with the numerous earlier attempts to have legislation passed, has been exhaustively explored by Donnison (1988). This chapter will set the scene for the rest of the book by exploring some of the features of maternity in Victorian England, and by considering the impact of the Midwives Act in the first ten years of its operation (although passed in 1902, it was not implemented until 1905 because of the time taken to develop the administrative apparatus to cope with issues such as having every midwife in the country identified and on a written Roll). Although the Act has been seen as a dividing line in the status and work of the midwife, this chapter will argue that it made very little difference to either the practice of midwives or the women's experience of maternity. A woman giving birth under the care of a midwife in 1914 would have had an experience that would have been recognised by her grandmother or great-grandmother in the previous century.

This chapter will also put the work and regulation of midwives into the broader context of contemporary debate around the health of the nation. There was concern that the health of the population was declining, particularly in urban areas, leading some commentators to argue that eugenic policies of selective breeding should be developed. It also resulted in a growing debate about the role of 'state medicine'; that is of government, at either local or national level, instigating and implementing policies designed to improve individual health through education and regulation.

Informing ideologies? Eugenics and physical deterioration

The 14 years between the opening of the twentieth century and the outbreak of the First World War have been characterised by historians as both a golden age, and a time of flux and uncertainty (Blom 2008). The impact of the Boer War in South Africa and the threat of German militarisation undoubtedly had an impact on how England saw herself. The self-confidence of the Victorian period when England was the world's first and pre-eminent industrial nation, with an Empire which stretched around the globe was increasingly tempered by concern about competition from other countries. In 1901, Arnold White, a radical writer on Imperial matters, wrote of the physical condition of army recruits. He claimed that in 1899 three-fifths of men volunteering for service in Manchester were rejected as being unfit (White 1901). Rowntree (1901) also discovered in his work on York that of 33,600 volunteers in York, Sheffield and Leeds between 1897 and 1900, the Army rejected 26.5 per cent as unfit, and accepted a further 29 per cent as 'specials', meaning that they barely passed muster for military service. It was Major General Sir John Maurice who perhaps had the biggest impact, however, with his article in 1902 in the *Contemporary Review*, a widely read periodical. He argued that:

> … taking into account those whom the officers did not think it worthwhile to bring before the Doctors, those whom the Doctors reject, and those who are rejected after trial in the Army, … to put it in its simplest terms, out of every five men who are willing to enlist, only two are fit to become efficient soldiers.
>
> (Maurice 1902)

Figures such as these profoundly shocked their middle-class readers. Haunted by the growing economic power and prestige of Germany in particular, and fearful of Britain 'losing her place in the sun' (a reference to the worldwide Empire Britain controlled), theorists and policy makers sought ways to arrest the perceived physical and moral decline of the population. One of the informing concerns was the decline in the birth rate among the middle classes. Completed family size had dropped dramatically by the end of the nineteenth century, yet the working classes were felt to be increasing at an undiminished rate. Steadman Jones (1984) highlighted the fears of the middle classes that cities in particular would be swamped by the 'unfit'. This concept came from 'eugenics', which had itself developed out of the popularising theories of evolution and the 'survival of the fittest' propounded in mid-century by Charles Darwin. Darwin's cousin, Francis Galton, who coined the term 'eugenic' in 1883, helped to develop a social theory of heredity (Farrell 1979). It was argued that humans could be divided into the 'fit' and 'unfit'; categories which roughly corresponded to social class. The professional middle classes, including many doctors, who were the main the supporters of eugenics or 'social Darwinism', believed that they were the guardians of the racial health of the nation. They were in favour of a meritocracy both mental and physical, which in practice meant the middle classes themselves. The working classes living in slum conditions were seen as obviously degenerate, as were the inbreeding, disease-ridden aristocracy (Jones 1980). Even capitalists were seen as contributing to what contemporaries described as 'race suicide' by employing, and therefore encouraging reproduction by, cheap 'unfit' labour for short-term gain.

Social Darwinism was a portmanteau of ideas which fed successfully on wider class fears about the falling birth rate, high infant mortality and the increasing visibility of the 'residuum': the very poor concentrated largely in urban centres. The importance of the debate on a political level was highlighted in 1904 with the creation and report of the Inter-departmental Committee on Physical Deterioration. This took as its term of reference the need '... to indicate generally the causes of such physical deterioration as does exist in certain classes' (HM Govt. 1904: v). Among its conclusions, the Committee suggested that 'there is no lack of evidence of increasing carelessness and deficient sense of responsibility among the younger women of the present day' (HM Govt. 1904: 55). The findings of the Committee did not support the thesis that the calibre of the British race was in inevitable decline. Instead it saw the problem of high infant mortality, for example, as caused not by innate systemic weakness but by ignorant mothers who were, it was hoped, amenable to education. The main recommendation of the Committee was centred around '... some great scheme of social education ...' aimed primarily at women (HM Govt. 1904: 57). Although overtly eugenic or Social Darwinist ideas were rejected by policy makers, the interaction between these ideas and questions of public health and sanitary reform were influential in the attempted development of state control over aspects of motherhood and the family (Davin 1978). Social hygiene and education for motherhood, for example, were seen as only applying to the working classes; and taught to them by members of the middle classes. Assistance in the form of health visitors or milk depot tokens included not only financial but moral means testing (Donzelot 1979). Personal and domestic hygiene, the feeding and care of infants, nutrition and the regulation of leisure activities, were all seen as legitimate areas of operation by those who distributed milk and maternity allowances. Acceptance of help implied at least a tacit acceptance of the moral codes of the instructors.

Not all commentators or policy makers subscribed to ideas of eugenics. After the Liberal victory in the general election of 1906, politicians such as Lloyd George and Churchill increasingly saw the way forward as being through social reform, which would at least give some support to the poorest in society. However, even legislation such as old age pensions embodied the basic early nineteenth-century Poor Law tenets of a difference between the 'deserving' and 'undeserving' poor. The former, who included pensioners, and those subject to cyclical unemployment were entitled to State help (Fraser 2003). The 'undeserving', who corresponded largely to the 'unfit' of eugenic thought, were the drunken, the workshy and the immoral, whose numbers included unmarried mothers. Concern about the health of the nation also reflected a growing interest in ideas of social responsibility, and of the duty of the wealthy to the poor. It has been argued that this strand of thought developed as a result of the growing power of the working classes through the trades union movement and the Labour Party, and of fear of revolution if grievances were not tackled (for the classic reading of the pre-war period as one of incipient revolution see Dangerfield 1935). For many it was, however, more than simply enlightened self-interest; women such as Rosalind Paget, an influential figure in attempts to professionalise midwifery, saw their role in terms of duty and responsibility and these were themes echoed by many others. This reflected not only concern about the health of the whole nation, but about the impact that poor living conditions and care had on individuals.

The Midwives Act, passed in 1902, was part of the drive to improve public health in England, both physically and morally, through the provision not only of large-scale works such as housing, sewerage and clean water, but through individual action. Midwives were increasingly seen by the government as part of this public health drive and the Midwives Act, and related legislation such as the Notification of Births Act (1907 and 1915), was both a symptom and cause of this development. Infant mortality in particular was repeatedly held up as an indictment on a civilised nation, and one which required immediate amelioration. Antenatal clinics, milk banks, mothercraft classes and baby clinics were all set up before the First World War in an attempt to tackle infant mortality rates. However, it has to be asked, to what extent midwives and mothers bought into this increasingly dominant ideology around individual action and responsibility, and what impact it had at the level of individual care?

Maternity care before 1900

In the nineteenth century most women in England were attended in labour by a midwife (Aveling 1872). This remained the case throughout the period despite debates about the encroachment of men into midwifery, the development of the new 'science' of obstetrics, or the sporadic founding of women's hospitals. However, the social landscape changed dramatically during the period, and this impacted significantly on midwifery.

Traditionally midwifery had been women's work, and evidence suggests that it was firmly rooted in the domestic sphere. Before the nineteenth century, women became midwives through an informal apprenticeship model by attending labours, particularly in the company of another midwife. There were textbooks available to women and evidence suggests that although the majority would have been illiterate, as was common for women of their time, many midwives were respectable and educated members of their communities (Hobby 1999). By the late eighteenth century men were carving out a niche for themselves in different medical fields, midwifery among them, and made financial and social capital by teaching and writing on their chosen speciality (Radcliffe 1967). Lectures were available in midwifery for both men and women, as were practical demonstrations; there is no evidence to suggest that they were taught differently (King 2007).

The concept of the 'take-over' of midwifery by men in the eighteenth and nineteenth centuries has occasioned much debate among historians

(Donnison 1988; Wilson 1995). It has to be seen in the context of the wider development of medicine, with the development of scientific and experimental enquiry, and in the light of the quintessential Victorian belief that things could be improved. For many doctors, their role was a mixture of status development and a genuine belief in doing the right thing. The career of James Aveling illustrated this well: as a young doctor he worked under James Simpson, and was an advocate of chloroform for childbirth; he went on to co-found a hospital for women in Sheffield, and in 1871 founded the Chelsea hospital for Women in London. The biographical sketch by Thornton (librarian of the Royal College of Obstetricians and Gynaecologists) in the 1967 reprint of Aveling's most famous book, *English Midwives: Their History and Prospects*, commented succinctly on the reasons for such a step: 'James Aveling decided that he must have a hospital appointment, and since he was too old for a junior position, and found it difficult to secure a senior one, he decided to found a new hospital for women' (Aveling 1967: xiv).

In a similar vein, hospitals were established for children and for particular areas of the body, such as Moorfields Eye Hospital which opened in 1802 (Granshaw 1989; Moscucci 1993). Medical journals were founded and doctors conducted long-running and sometimes bitter disputes about methods of care and treatment (*The Lancet*, still one of the most widely read medical journals in the world, was founded in 1823). The holy grail for anyone involved in midwifery was the saving of maternal and infant lives, and one of the most famous, and long-running, disputes among doctors who practised midwifery was the acceptability or otherwise of Caesarean sections (Radford 1880). Despite this, hospitals for women were not intended as places for babies to be born; Aveling, in his prospectus for his proposed hospital in Sheffield, explained why:

> Women are to be attended when in labour at their own homes. The earlier lying-in hospitals adopted a different plan to this. They took into hospital all cases, whether they were natural or unnatural … it was found that when puerperal fever broke out, that it spread from bed to bed with such fatal rapidity and with such awful results that the building often had to be shut up for a season, and thus the benefits of the charities were interrupted and defeated.
>
> (*Sheffield and Rotherham Independent* 12.12.1863)

He was not exaggerating; even Florence Nightingale, the pioneer of nursing, had to close her supposedly 'model' lying-in hospital in London when fever swept through the building in 1867, killing many new mothers (Mathers and McIntosh 2000).

Women's hospitals did have in-patient beds, but they were designed for those suffering from disease or trauma. Many of the early operations conducted were concerned with repairing the damage caused by prolonged years of reproduction, difficult births and ill-nourished bodies: 'I was in labour thirty-six hours and after all that suffering had to be delivered by instruments, and was ruptured too badly to have anything done to help me. I am still suffering from the ill-effects today. This is thirty-one years ago' (Llewelyn Davies 1915: 70). Records from the Sheffield Hospital demonstrate that such long-standing cases were not unusual, with many women in their 50s and 60s receiving treatment for injuries they had sustained giving birth 20 or 30 years previously. It was only after suffering for so long with prolapsed wombs, ruptured perineums or fistulas, that surgical and anaesthetic techniques developed to the point where interventions might have a chance of success.

Doctors were at this point, whatever their speciality, men. Although the Royal College of Physicians had been founded in 1518, their work did not include the use of instruments and they did not perform surgery. Early nineteenth-century efforts to improve the social status and remuneration of surgeons were slow to gather momentum. The image remained in the public mind of barber- or butcher-surgeons, who, as far as midwifery was concerned, were called in with instruments such as forceps or a craniotomy hook, when all else had failed. The famous illustration of a man-midwife sums up this dichotomy by contrasting the forceps and hooks of the man with the domestic para-phernalia of the woman. In their efforts to create a closed shop, whereby they controlled medical education, entry and practice, doctors created the template for what sociologists have seen as creating a 'profession' (Arney 1982). Within this the practice of midwifery was still seen as suspect by many doctors; it was not mentioned at all in the 1858 Act of Parliament designed to regulate the practice of medicine, and not until 1886 did the General Medical Council (the governing body of doctors) require any kind of qualification in midwifery for doctors. This was partly because it was associated with surgery which continued to lag behind physics in terms of status, and partly because it was primarily done by non-specialist doctors who worked in domestic settings rather than hospitals. Those who did specialise in midwifery were therefore of necessity robust in their defence of their area of expertise and their belief that it was equal to any other branch of medicine. Given that midwifery had always been part of social rather than medical discourse, the defence of doctors relied heavily on distancing themselves from female midwives who exemplified the domestic role of midwifery, and in placing their work on a rational scientific footing. Loudon (1986) argued that doctors' education as far as midwifery was concerned probably declined in quality over the nineteenth century, and that there were no scientific breakthroughs which made birth safer or more pleasant for mothers or their offspring. The major advances in midwifery centred around pain relief and antiseptics, both of which were developed through other specialities, and were not widely available to women even at the end of the nineteenth century.

Deliberately or otherwise, doctors seeking to gain a foothold in the lying-in room were extremely scathing of midwives, who were both their competition and the millstone around their necks in terms of a professional project. As Towler and Bramall (1986) commented, however, that although there were many vicious things written by doctors about midwives, the quality of actual relationships probably varied enormously. Doctors such as Aveling could afford to be rude about midwives, but doctors working in single-handed practices in towns and rural areas were probably more accommodating. Midwifery was laborious work, and evidence for the twentieth century, where doctors and midwives might have extremely close working relationships, was probably equally true of the nineteenth. In 1869 it was claimed in a Survey by the London Obstetrical Society that the majority of poor women were delivered by midwives, regardless of whether they lived in rural or urban areas. However, in fashionable and wealthy areas such as the West End of London, less than 2 per cent of births were attended by midwives (Aveling 1872: 164). By the late nineteenth century it was fashionable to be cared for, and delivered by, a doctor; probably a reflection of the status symbol effect of the cost rather than particular ideas about improved safety (Jalland 1988).

Partly related to her work, which was increasingly plied among the poorer sections of society, the image of the midwife which has resonated down the years has been that of Charles Dickens' Sarah Gamp, mentioned by every history of midwifery and nursing as shorthand for the idea of a midwife. Dickens' influence was clearly wide and the 'Gamp' became part of colloquial language; commenting on her practice in the 1930s, midwife Alice Pearson described her untrained competition as 'Gamps' (interview). This image of the midwife as dirty, ignorant, drunken and slipshod was promulgated by many doctors. Aveling wrote in 1872 of midwives as 'ignorant and often dissipated' who were to blame for maternal death and the subsequent break-up of the family home (1872: 169–70). Sarah Gamp was also, Heagerty (1996) argued, taken as the mould from which all lay midwives were formed according to the middle-class leaders of the Midwives Institute. This group of largely middle-class women were to become very influential in the pressure for a Midwives Act and beyond, and their view of working-class midwifery helped to shape discourse about the role well into the twentieth century.

Much of the criticism of midwives hinged around doctors' beliefs that midwifery should be practised only by themselves, but a potent strand of critical writing on midwifery came from those who wanted to secure education and training for midwives. Although there had been some Church licensing of midwives in earlier centuries, by the nineteenth century this system had fallen into abeyance, and only a woman and her peers could decide if she was a midwife or not. Not all women who cared for women in labour necessarily described themselves as midwives which makes it very hard for historians to generalise about the type of woman who practised midwifery, let alone her level of skill or knowledge (McIntosh 1998). Evidence from Sheffield suggested that even midwives who had some basic training through the Hospital for Women did not earn a living wage; the average annual caseload was 73, with fees of three to five shillings per case. This gave an annual wage of £20 in 1900; high compared to many other midwives, but not a living wage at a time when skilled male workers had an average income of £100 per year. In 1881,

17 midwives advertised their services through the *Sheffield Trade Directory*; implying they were professional midwives in the sense that they saw it as an occupation rather than a neighbourly service. The youngest woman mentioned in the *Directory* was Elizabeth Jarvis who was 35, and the oldest was Eliza Broadhurst who was 63. All of the women who advertised themselves were married or widowed, and the majority had older working children at home, according to the relevant census data. Their husbands tended to do skilled work in the light metal trades for which Sheffield was famous. Even amongst this select group of midwives, five did not describe themselves as being midwives in the census taken in the same year. Only Elizabeth Jarvis was still advertising herself as a midwife ten years later; the turnover of midwives advertising in annual trade directories was such that even for these women it was a choice of employment based on economic need and lifestyle rather than conviction (McIntosh 1998). In Nottingham, one woman who lived in the village of Lambley before the First World War remembered 'Aunt Sarah' who was called the midwife because she helped when babies came and '... laying out an' sitting up with people all night and that sort of thing'.

There were sporadic attempts to develop midwifery training and regulation in the nineteenth century, with the running being made by doctors, who wanted midwives to do the bulk of tedious normal domiciliary midwifery under the auspices of a hospital. Although the majority of midwives remained untrained, those who did seek training had to do so under the umbrella of one of the women's hospitals scattered across the country. General hospitals usually had space for, and treated, many more men than women. They also refused to admit pregnant women or their offspring:

> ... no woman big with child, no Child under six years of Age (except in urgent or particular cases, such as fractures, cutting for the stone, amputations, couching, trepanning, or where some other surgical operation may be required) ... to be admitted as in-patients.
>
> (*Sheffield Royal Infirmary Annual Report* 1813)

The loopholes were obviously many, and admittance of children and pregnant women was probably not that uncommon, however discouraged it was officially; the list of expectations covers most of the procedures a hospital would be attempting during the nineteenth century.

Midwifery trainees did their deliveries in the district and once qualified continued to work there. Aveling, a driving force behind the campaign for midwifery education and registration, was very clear about the reasons for instituting training:

> In Sheffield we have a few able midwives, who understand their business well and prove themselves sources of comfort to many poor sufferers; but we also have a larger class, pretentious and ignorant, causing grief and misery ... the ignorance met with among midwives in this town is notorious to medical men
>
> (*Sheffield Independent* 12.12.1863)

The Sheffield Hospital for Women required its trainees to attend 30 labours and births, and to concentrate only on the 'natural'. What constituted a natural labour or delivery is not discussed in the surviving records, but the use of the word marked clearly that cases were to be ring fenced as either for doctors or for midwives. A similar concept was promulgated in contemporary textbooks:

> Finally, any training which the midwife receives should not encourage her to undertake cases which are out of her sphere, since by doing so she will incur a very grave responsibility, but should rather impress upon her the importance of sending for medical help when any unnatural condition exists or is threatening.
>
> (Donald 1894: 2)

This idea is one which has echoed down through the twentieth century and is, in essence, still to be found in the legal responsibilities of contemporary midwives (NMC 2004). What constituted 'natural' in the context of pregnancy and birth has never been a constant; it is a social as much as a biological construct; but the conduct of such labours has continued to be something that midwives have fought for, an artificial distinction perhaps not appreciated by women.

None of this is to exaggerate developments in maternity care during the nineteenth century. The majority of women continued to be delivered in their own homes by locally based midwives. For these midwives their work was an extension of their female role, rooted in domesticity, and one which was dependant on the life cycle of the individual; midwives were never young or single, but had children of their own and were either married or widowed. It is unlikely that they saw themselves as engaged in a profession, vocation, or even craft, any more than they would have characterised taking in lodgers or washing in similar terms. Such a role was, however, under increasing threat from campaigners, whether middle-class women searching for a professional outlet; doctors attempting to stake their claim to posterity; or politicians increasingly anxious about the toll of infant mortality and morbidity on the country's military strength.

Delivering maternity care in 1902

In the years between 1900 and 1914 motherhood was elevated to the status of an almost religious vocation, with ideas of 'duty' and 'sacrifice' abounding in any discussion of mothers. Speaking at the London Conference on Infant Mortality in 1906, John Burns, President of the Local Government Board (forerunner of the Ministry of Health) famously commented that people should 'glorify, dignify and purify motherhood; for what the mother is, the children will be' (McIntosh 1997). To this end, mothers could be, and were, vilified for not taking what was considered to be proper care of their infants. There was in this period, however, no reciprocal focus on the health of the mother or on her care during pregnancy or birth. Antenatal care, where it did sporadically develop, was for the welfare of the unborn child, not its mother, and postnatal care did not exist.

The concept of infant welfare was a specific one which grew out of national concerns for the perceived declining physical health of the nation. It was primarily developed, however, by practitioners rather than theorists, and was pragmatic in idea and execution. The main influences on its development were George McCleary, the Medical Officer of Health (MoH) for Battersea; George Newman who did the same role in Finsbury and later worked for the Board of Education and the Ministry of Health; and Arthur Newsholme who was the MoH for Brighton and was then an officer at the Local Government Board (Newman 1906; McCleary 1935; Newsholme 1935, 1936). All three developed local schemes around aspects of maternal and infant welfare in the pre-war period, and all three went on to have considerable influence over national debate and policy formation. As a result of their health roles within local government, they and other MoHs were generally pragmatic about what could be achieved through public initiatives. The role of MoH had developed in the mid-nineteenth century, and was codified under the Public Health Act of 1872. The post was filled initially by generalist doctors, but became increasingly specialised, and at the same time influential and far reaching within specific communities. The MoH had responsibility for everything from housing and public sanitation, to abattoirs and food quality. By 1914 they were, in many areas, running infant welfare clinics, milk banks and mothercraft classes through their local health departments, as the maternal and infant welfare movement began to gather steam. These measures were designed to address the problem of stubbornly high rates of infant mortality in the face of falling general death rates. To a certain extent there were concerns about racial decline embedded in these initiatives; one contributor to the *Journal of the Royal Sanitary Institute*, to which MoHs belonged, argued in 1908 that:

> While it is urgently necessary that the question of better housing, better milk supply, the economic position of mothers, and the education of mothers still receive immediate attention, it is also necessary to realise that while criminals, inebriates and the feeble-minded continue to propagate, successful efforts in lowering the death rate among children of such parents must lead to racial degeneracy.
>
> (*Journal of the Royal Sanitary Institute* 2: 758–62)

This was undoubtedly the underlying belief of many, but was tempered by the views of writers such as Newsholme who, in looking back on his career, commented that even education through health visitors and mothercraft classes was not as significant to infant and maternal life as material provision such as medical care, or clean milk and water supplies (Newsholme 1935).

Classes, both municipal and voluntary, developed to educate working-class mothers on every aspect of infant rearing. The Motherhood League in Sheffield for example, had by 1909, a rolling programme of eight public lectures on topics such as care of babies in health, food values and what to buy, and the clothing of children (McIntosh 1997). One lecture in the series covered pregnancy, but nothing was said about birth. With very few books of advice available, assuming women had the time or education to read them, it is clear that information around pregnancy and birth must have been local and community or family based. It is very difficult even to be certain about exactly who delivered babies in 1902. Women had a choice of specialists, general practitioners, midwives – trained or untrained – or neighbours, and there was no official paper work to be completed which would have specified the person involved. Sometimes the situation could be downright misleading; a doctor might be engaged to take a case but that did not necessarily mean that he would deliver the baby or even be present at its birth. Labour could be a tedious affair and doctors might work with a midwife who would do the bulk of the care and call him out if either she or the family felt it necessary.

Whoever they chose for their care, evidence suggests that women, both rich and poor, were quite opinionated about their doctors and midwives. One of the richest sources of information around women's experience of maternity in this period comes from a collection of letters gathered by the Women's Co-operative Guild, a campaigning organisation of some 32,000 working-class women, and originally published in 1915 (Llewelyn Davies). These women, who were associated with the Co-operative movement, were by no means the lowest of the low, but their stories give powerful voice to those whose stories are very seldom told: ordinary working-class women, and particularly around a subject such as maternity which tends to be hidden from many mainstream histories. As well as detailing hardship and suffering, the letters also provide evidence to suggest that even in this period women were not cowed by medical authority and very much had their own ideas about the experiences and care they wanted during childbirth. To a certain extent these letters do have to be read as forming part of a larger political project; the Guild campaigned tirelessly for maternal and child welfare projects, including in the inter-war years, hospitals for birth and the wider provision of contraception (Lewis 1980). The Guild also supported the training of midwives, and many of its members who contributed letters had plenty to say about ignorant midwives, and indeed, ignorant doctors. This does suggest that even working-class women did not necessarily see themselves as from the same social milieu as midwives; those midwives who were not trained were not generally seen as repositories of kindness and wisdom, but as potentially as dangerous and ignorant as some doctors and politicians suggested they were.

Working-class women in Llewelyn Davies' collection talked about putting themselves in the hands of a 'good doctor' and of saving money towards this (Llewelyn Davies 1915: 92). They were also aware of the role of the doctor in attending emergencies, and the drama engendered by his attendance; one mother commented that 'Instruments had to be used, and I heard the doctor say he could not tell whether my life could be saved or not' (Llewelyn Davies 1915: 31). However, there was no remembered sense of deference; one woman complained about doctors arguing over the best management of a case (Llewelyn Davies 1915: 84) whilst another one complained about the doctor not coming (Llewelyn Davies 1915: 67). One woman believed that a doctor caused her to be very ill through 'hurrying the birth, instead of giving nature a chance' (Llewelyn Davies 1915: 122), a charge supported by the historian Loudon (1992) who argued that 'family' doctors were often tempted to hurry births with chloroform and forceps because their workload was so high.

It is likely that the majority of births in England were still attended solely by a midwife, whether she described herself as such or not, and in fact not needing a doctor might be equated in the woman's mind with her own health and stamina: 'During my labour I was never bad more than about three or four hours. I felt I could get out of bed the first day, and I never had the doctor, only an old midwife' (Llewelyn Davies 1915: 26). However, even poor women could be scathing about the quality of care they received from midwives: one claimed that her midwife had missed a twin pregnancy during a miscarriage at three or four months and the woman, thinking she was no longer pregnant was amazed to give birth. Of the midwife she commented, '[she] was no doubt all right when things were straightforward' but she argued that:

Now if I had been able to have a qualified midwife when I had the miscarriage, we should have known there was another child, and I could have been medically treated, all that suffering could have been prevented, and I might have had a strong child.

(Llewelyn Davies 1915: 34–35)

There are a multiplicity of concepts implicit in this statement; the mother did not feel it was her responsibility to know that she was still pregnant, but rather she wanted and expected a 'professional' to be able to tell her. Furthermore, she believed that if it had been known that she was pregnant, she would have received care that would have ensured a favourable outcome, although, in fact, neither doctors nor midwives were able to offer such care at that period. Women were also not averse to making choices about their care: 'when I was pregnant the second time, I heard that the midwife I had the first time had started drinking, so I was afraid to have her. I had a doctor and it was as well I had, as I did not go on as well as I did the first time' (Llewelyn Davies 1915: 36). In writing of their midwives women were aware that they often filled a multiplicity of roles which might impact on the care they were able to give. One woman commented with evident resentment that the midwife at her second birth 'having lodgers to attend to left him unwashed for an hour after his birth. She never troubled to get his lungs inflated, and he was two days without crying. I had no doctor' (Llewelyn Davies 1915: 31). Census returns from places such as Sheffield indicate clearly that particularly in areas of heavy industry where there was no tradition of women working in skilled trades, they did combine work such as midwifery and taking in lodgers in order to make a living wage (McIntosh 1997). Doctors were more expensive than midwives, and therefore the implication was that you got what you could pay for. As one woman commented: 'I had to depend on my neighbours for what help they could give me during labour and the lying in period'; this sounds to have been through necessity rather than choice, but is a reminder of the domestic nature of birth at this time (Llewelyn Davies 1915: 24). The idea of community for information and support was clearly an important one as several women talked of moving and giving birth in a place where they knew no one, including the midwife: 'My last [birth] was the worst; we had removed away to a strange place, and I happened to get a woman who did not know her work' (Llewelyn Davies 1915: 83, see also 102 and 112).

At the other end of the social spectrum, Jalland (1988) explored the domestic lives of women in political families in the late nineteenth and early twentieth century, primarily through their personal letters and diaries. For them as much as their working-class counterparts, biology was very much destiny, with pregnancy, birth and child-rearing taking centre stage in their lives, no matter how wealthy or politically connected they were. Even the wealthy women discussed by Jalland relied on a network of family and friends for advice and support. She commented that although this period was seen as transitional in terms of the movement of birth from domestic to medical event, for this social class, doctors when they did attend appear to have arrived on the scene as late as possible, and their advice was often ignored or contradicted by women. During a difficult labour in 1908 one woman was told by her doctor that the birth would be delayed if she took chloroform; she decided to have the drug regardless (Jalland 1988: 148). In their letters to friends and relatives women discussed the merits of different doctors and different techniques such as the application of forceps and the best time to suture a perineum; implying that experience was pooled and knowledge could be quite detailed (Jalland 1988: 149). This suggests that whatever doctors' beliefs in their own powers and expertise, in the period around 1902 women of all classes exercised a significant degree of choice and control over their experience of childbirth.

Interestingly husbands were not necessarily excluded from the debate and the process. The letters to the Women's Co-op Guild make clear that this could cut both ways, with both cruel and generous loving husbands written about. One woman wrote of being in labour with her fifth child whilst her husband lay very ill in the other room. She commented that 'I dare not let my husband in his precarious condition hear a cry of pain from me, and travail [labour] pain cannot always be stifled; and here again the doctor helped me by giving me a sleeping draught to administer to him as soon as I felt the pangs of childbirth' (Llewelyn Davies 1915: 47). Note that it was the husband who received a sleeping draught, rather than the labouring woman who received anything for her pain! The same solicitude for her husband is recorded by Edith Lyttelton whose husband had lost his first wife to child-birth. She refused to use chloroform in spite of her doctor 'begging' her to let the doctors use it. Her reasoning was that she had heard women often screamed under the influence of chloroform and she did not want to put her husband through that anxiety (Jalland 1988: 147). Husbands certainly seem to have been in close proximity when their wives were labouring, and many were with their wives offering what was clearly significant support (Jalland 1988: 145) As Jalland argued, this suggested a high level of emotional intimacy in many of these marriages; childbirth although still domestic was not exclusively female. Similarly for respondents to Llewelyn Davies, a good or bad husband impacted significantly on the experience of maternity, and women wrote of the importance of their partners: 'I am very pleased to say that, having one of the best of all husbands, I suffered nothing during pregnancy ...' (Llewelyn Davies 1915: 142), but others wrote of husbands who drank and demanded sex immediately after the baby was born and the suffering which this caused both physically and emotionally (Llewelyn Davies 1915: 49).

The vast majority of women delivered at home. Clearly the type of space available depended very much on the family circumstances: 'Naturally the midwife must make the best of the houses in which her work lies; the more unhygienic, the dustier and the dirtier the houses, the greater will be the risk of infection ...' wrote one doctor in his textbook for midwives (Fairbairn 1914: 108). Some women laboured and delivered in the one room where the rest of their family lived, with no light, warmth or privacy. Fairbairn's book of instructions to midwives detailed the need for scrupulous cleanliness including the removal of most of the furniture and the provision of clean clothes and bedding. He accepted, however, that '... among the poor, the mid-wife must make use of what the patient can provide' (Fairbairn 1914: 112). Even for wealthy women delivery at home was the norm, often with a monthly nurse available for the birth and the lying-in period.

Lying-in hospitals were charitable institutions used by a few; principally the wives of skilled workers who paid for the hospital through subscriptions. The very destitute delivered in the workhouse, although by 1902 this held few of the horrors of 50 years previously. Poor Law hospitals were run separately from the rest of the workhouse, usually in separate buildings, and the care they gave was equal to that of the private lying-in hospitals. Midwives were trained in workhouse hospitals and the office of parish doctor was a popular and remunerative appointment. Care was, however, little different to that offered at home with pain relief not freely available and operations such as the Caesarean used very infrequently. In Liverpool the first Caesarean was not performed until 1894, and even in Manchester where several pro-Caesarean doctors lived and worked the numbers of Caesarean performed each year did not reach double figures until 1902 (Towler and Bramall 1986: 153). Only gradually were the memories of the nineteenth-century terrors of hospital birth fading, when fever sweeping through the wards could leave in its wake a huge loss of life. The gradual acceptance of ideas of antisepsis and asepsis contributed to a reduction in these sudden losses of life and the concomitant wariness about hospital delivery (Wootton 2007). Hospital birth remained, however, very much outside the experience of most women.

Women would be very unlikely to receive any antenatal care, and would only call the doctor or midwife once in labour. Even estimating the due date might be hit-and-miss as a missed period in a malnourished woman would not necessarily signal pregnancy. For many women there was doubt until they felt the baby move at about 16 to 18 weeks of pregnancy; that is to say nearly half way through its typical length. If a miscarriage was threatened then bed rest was prescribed, although this type of advice seems to have come from friends as much as from medical men (Jalland 1988). Other than that pregnancy and birth were regarded as normal life events and women took pride in continuing with their daily routines until labour; writing in 1906 Molly Trevelyan detailed her social life and charity work as well as many miles of walking without giving any particular indication that she was pregnant (Jalland 1988: 138). After birth many wealthy women hired monthly nurses, to care for themselves and their babies. These might be women who in other circumstances would act as midwives; in many cases they worked in tandem with doctors and actually delivered the baby. For working-class women the quality of postnatal care they received goes some way to explaining why untrained midwives continued to be a popular choice. It was not just a question of their affordability (a midwife would charge about 4 shillings compared to a doctor whose fee would be one or two pounds); they offered significant domestic help post-natally including childcare, washing and the preparation of meals, allowing the new mother to have some relief from domestic chores. The one thing which they did not seem to have done – and which trained midwives were later encouraged to do – was to wash the woman. 'For a whole week we were obliged to lie on clothes stiff and stained, and the stench under the clothes was abominable, and added to this we were commanded to keep the babies under the clothes' (Llewelyn Davies 1915: 32). But these midwives were from the same social sphere as the women they cared for and would not have complained about patched clothes, less than pristine sheets or crowded living conditions. Women did not have to put on a front for their midwives. As the LGB Report into the 1902 Midwives Act observed, '... in many cases women prefer the old type of attendants, who is probably well known to them and is usually more helpful in the house although she is often uncleanly and inexpert' (LGB 1909: 5). One textbook, written for midwives in 1893, described the continuing existence of a neighbourhood idea of birth which went right back to medieval times and beyond: 'In poor houses it is not uncommon for anxious or curious relatives and neighbours to crowd in. In such cases one woman may be allowed to remain to act as assistant, but the others must be asked to retire' (Donald 1894: 80).

The domestic, rather than medical role played by midwives was clearly hugely significant to the women who used their services, and was underlined by respondents to the Women's Co-operative Guild survey. One woman explained that problems were caused by midwives being too busy and not attending properly to the care of mothers: 'What is really wanted is a supply of real good midwives who could be got for a month to see to all require-ments of the patient and the home while the woman has a fair chance of recovering' (Llewelyn Davies 1915: 86). It is perhaps no surprise, for women struggling to pay even their neighbourhood midwife to attend for a few days that some began to look to hospital care after birth as a break from domestic drudgery as 'there is no peace for the wife at home' (Llewelyn Davies 1915: 89). In the inter-war period this feeling was to become an increasingly influential one in the design and execution of maternity care.

Birth and death

By the beginning of the twentieth century it appeared that the terrible rates of maternal death seen up to the 1880s had finally begun to decline for good. The introduction, and increasing use of, antiseptics in midwifery meant that puerperal fever became less of a scourge. The cause and source of the fever was still unknown, and it was uniquely feared because it killed women in the days after what might be an uneventful miscarriage or birth. Except for cleanliness there seemed to be no way to tackle it. It was particularly prevalent in areas where there were many births, particularly the lying-in hospitals which had developed sporadically in the mid-Victorian years and where in some cases over 80 per cent of in-patient deaths were due to fever (Loudon 1992: 200). The safest place to give birth at the beginning of the twentieth century was still at home, and few doctors seriously questioned this hegemony. As Loudon (1992) observed, however, maternal mortality did not follow a linear downward path; in 1893, the maternal mortality rate was 65.1 deaths per 10,000 maternities and although by 1910 this had fallen to 35.5, it crept back up to 41.7 by 1914.

Despite the maternal death rate, women, midwives and doctors did not explicitly use the language of risk in 1902. The uncertainty and possible danger surrounding pregnancy, labour and the puerperium were, however, a central part of how women viewed their lives, regardless of age or class:

> I do not think I was very different in my pregnancies to others. I always prepared myself to die, and I think this awful depression is common to most at this time. And when bothered by several other children, and not knowing how to make ends meet, death in some cases would be welcome if it were not the dread of the children. How would they get on without their mother?
>
> (Llewelyn Davies 1915: 166)

Blodgett's work on female diarists suggests that pregnancy and birth were times of excitement, competition and deep fear (1989). They were to women what battlefields were for men, and the likelihood of suffering, not to mention the possibility of death was seen as necessary and character building. Some writers have suggested that pain completed an aristocratic woman's sense of womanhood and duty. Margot Asquith wrote in 1916 that to eliminate the pain of childbirth 'would take too much drama out of life' (Jalland 1988: 175). Jalland drew attention to the fears of these wealthy and well-connected women when faced with pregnancy. One woman described her friend as having been 'dreadfully ill and nearly died on the journey down from Scotland … I must say I think her pluck is wonderful. I'm sure I wouldn't face it again if I had been as near dying as she was when she had that last stillborn baby' (Jalland 1988: 164). Mary, the daughter of British Prime Minister Gladstone, nearly died after an incomplete miscarriage in 1886 followed by peritonitis, despite the attentions of a swathe of doctors and a medical bill of £235 (Jalland 1988: 166). The loss of a baby or mother was not uncommon, and women made wills in their pregnancies. Blame was not easy to apportion; Laura Tennant died in 1886 following the delivery of a nine-pound baby whose birth required 'an hour's work with instruments' according to her sister-in-law, and was followed by 'a horrid unusual haemorrhage' (Jalland 1988: 178). The doctors insisted that her illness and death eight days later was due to 'a very bad liver illness and nothing to do with confinement'. It was not only the wealthy who suffered; Alice Hartley, a working-class woman living in the East End of Sheffield died 23 days after the normal birth of a healthy baby in May 1910. When six days after the birth Alice complained of feeling ill, the midwife who attended her, 76-year-old Charlotte Ransom, suggested that it was caused by eating cake too soon after delivery. Not until three days later did Alice's doctor put in an appearance from his surgery on the other side of the city. He began treating her for pneumonia, having failed to take her temperature because he had smashed his thermometer. Alice died of puerperal fever, in a case that reflected badly on all concerned (Mathers and McIntosh 2000: 47).

The Midwives Act, passed in 1902 and enacted in 1905, was designed to stop such ignorance and muddle, at least on the part of midwives. It was described as providing for the registration of midwives, but it was far more wide reaching than that. It provided for the annual publication of the names of all those midwives currently in practice: the Midwives Roll. It also included strictures about the types of woman who could appear on the Roll, and minimum standards for training. The area which has caused most controversy for historians is that of statutory supervision which was laid down by the Act. Heagerty argued that supervision was a way of controlling midwives; punishing those who, for whatever reason, were considered to be unacceptable by those who controlled midwifery. After 1905, when the Act came into force, no midwife could practise without being on the Roll, and therefore, as Heagerty termed it, 'registered with the state' (1996). She argued that the Act led to a very narrow definition of the scope of the role of midwife and put what had been a local neighbourhood craft in the hands of a powerful elite. Heagerty suggested that the middle-class women who made up the membership of the Midwives Institute and whom, as we have seen, campaigned for a midwifery act, knew nothing of how ordinary midwives practised. Taking their cue from wider concerns about national deterioration, they sought to inculcate working-class midwives with ideas about cleanliness, respectability and the willingness to be subordinate to the medical profession. Hannam (1997) argued that Heagerty's thesis was too narrow and too reductionist, although she admitted that such ideas as demonstrating moral character to their working-class clients were of central importance to leaders of the Midwives Institute. Clearly, in order for these middle-class ideas to be assimilated and promulgated, the best option would be for only those midwives who had undergone training, and could be expected therefore to adhere to the rules, to practise.

However, the government recognised that this would be completely impractical since very few midwives possessed any training. Without allowing untrained midwives to continue practising there would simply not have been enough midwives available to deliver the babies. Until 1910, therefore, all lay midwives could continue to practise. Thereafter only trained midwives and '*bona fides*' could attend births 'habitually and for gain'. *Bona fides* were those who were considered to be of sufficient local standing and expertise to continue in practice. As they retired, however, they would be replaced with trained and qualified midwives. In this way the regulated entry of a profession seemed to be developing, controlled by education and registration. It was hoped that 'handywomen' – untrained midwives who were seen by the authorities as very much in the Sarah Gamp mould – would gracefully disappear from the scene after 1905, a belief that proved to be somewhat optimistic. Evidence suggests that the Act did not change who midwives were or how they operated; neither did it lead to an atmosphere of hostility between beleaguered working-class midwives and their clients on the one hand, and their middle-class tormentors on the other. Untrained married and widowed midwives continued to ply their trade in their local communities (Heagerty 1990; McIntosh 2000). It was estimated, for example, that in Rotherham in 1907–8 a quarter of births were still attended by handywomen, and the Medical Officer of Health in Sheffield suggested that there were still 30 handywomen in practice in the city in 1909. The practice of the handywoman 'habitually and for gain' (as opposed to in an emergency) was explicitly prohibited after 1910, but evidence suggested that they continued to operate, often under the wing of local GPs, until well into the 1930s. One woman, who was an active member of the Women's Co-operative Guild and worked as a maternity nurse under several GPs, remembered that they lent her books and taught her to use forceps 'which midwives were not taught in hospital'. Despite being unable to afford to train as a midwife, she clearly felt supported and respected by the doctors with whom she worked (Llewelyn Davies 1931: 44).

However, as Heagerty (1996) argued, the creation of the Central Midwives Board (CMB) which was to be the regulatory body for midwifery in England and Wales, and which was made up of medical, midwifery and lay elites, was used to control and punish those midwives who did not fit the 'ideal'. She suggested that local supervisors of midwives, usually lay people, could not distinguish between dangerous practice and the exigencies of caring for under-nourished women in poor conditions. Evidence from local studies does not suggest an over-arching project, however, but rather that supervision was interoperated differently in different areas, and could range from overtly punitive to largely supportive and enabling (Davies 1988; Mottram 1997; McIntosh 1998). As we have seen, many midwives did not describe themselves as midwives, and there is no evidence that the majority of them had a sense of self as workers, never mind as potentially part of a broader professional project. Researchers on midwifery in the USA and in Britain have argued that legislation such as the Sheppard-Towner Act in the USA, and the 1902 Act in England and Wales, downgraded traditional skills in favour of a medicalised, scientific approach to childbirth (Donnison 1988; Ladd-Taylor 1988; Heagerty 1990). However, the reality seems to have been that midwives had very little sense of themselves as a cohesive group, never mind one which possessed a developed set of skills or beliefs about practice.

That is not to say that the Act did not divide midwives, particularly since they were in competition with doctors and increasingly with hospitals and maternity homes for a declining number of births. Reagan (1995) argued that in the USA midwives hastened their own professional demise by failing to act cohesively. In England there were stories of midwives having each other prosecuted, or referred to the CMB, presumably in an attempt to drive out competition. The willingness of one midwife in Sheffield to have another prosecuted in 1906 for the alleged supply of diachylon, a lead-based abortifacient, bears this out (McIntosh 1998). Certainly, as Heagerty (1996) suggested, trained midwives had little time for the others on the Roll, with many insisting that the inclusion of *bona fides* was an insult. One of the new breed of trained midwives complained that local handywomen were 'old women, absolutely ignorant, very dirty and exceedingly drunk'; a classic 'Sarah Gamp' picture (McIntosh 1998). Needless to say handywomen responded, accusing young unmarried midwives as having no knowledge or experience, and getting all their information from books alone. The same midwife also highlighted tensions between local doctors and trained midwives, suggesting that one GP accused midwives such as herself of being 'scantily qualified practitioners' who were taking cases and fees that rightly belonged to GPs (McIntosh 1998). These tensions were caused by competition between doctors, various types of midwifery practitioners, and hospitals for a share of a declining pool of births. At a time when everyone was paid per case, the loss of one or two to a rival could mean a very significant drop in income, particularly for midwives whom, as we have seen, struggled to make anything like a living wage. Local studies have suggested that it was these economic realities, rather than conspiracies around the deliberate destruction of working-class midwives by an educated, urban elite, which caused tensions within midwifery after 1902.

In the first ten years of its operation the biggest difference made by the Midwives Act to maternity care seems to have been in the changing attitude of doctors, public health officials and government to the women who delivered babies. Prior to the Act, midwives were assumed to be responsible for the majority of puerperal fever cases; these were caused by a streptococcal wound infection which led to 35–50 per cent of maternal deaths. In 1896, the MoH for Sheffield complained in his Annual Report that midwives were 'wholly uneducated and ignorant of the first principals of cleanliness and methods of preventing this disease'. By 1907, two years after the implementation of the Act, the right it gave to take punitive action against midwives was demonstrated:

> 46 cases of puerperal fever were notified, in 21 of which the confinement was attended by a midwife. In each of the latter cases arrangements were made for the midwife to have disinfectant baths, and for the disinfection of her clothes and outfit. In each case the possible origin of the disease was investigated and the midwife was temporarily suspended from practice.
>
> (*MoH Report Sheffield* 1907: 42)

Suspension of practice meant loss of income, as well as the possible stigma of local authority ministrations. Doctors received no such attention despite being responsible for the majority of puerperal fever cases in Sheffield that year. Beyond the spectre of discipline, however, local medical officials began to use different language when talking to and about midwives in the years after 1902. As the Mayor of Sheffield commented when addressing the city's midwives in 1906, they should possess 'a high idea of their calling, and endeavour to exercise an educational influence wherever they went' (McIntosh 1998: 418, for other examples of the use of this style of language, see Dove 1985). Midwives were being co-opted into wider plans for health, and conceived as potential 'missionaries' in the spread of ideas concerning health and hygiene to women. Furthermore they were being rehabilitated in language which carried overtly religious overtones. Interestingly the Health Department did not distinguish between trained and *bona fide* midwives, but appropriated them all as potential proselytisers.

The need for trained midwives meant a concomitant requirement for training schools. Although midwives continued to receive the majority of their training by following qualified midwives giving care in women's homes, it was increasingly recognised by both providers of midwifery and medical training, that the easiest way to deal with growing numbers of recruits was to train them in an institutional setting. This chimed with the growing acceptability of hospital birth to women, both in terms of its perceived safety in comparison with the records of Victorian lying-in hospitals, but also in the greater availability of pain relief in the institutional as opposed to the domestic setting (Pitcock and Clark 1992). Debates over the place of birth would intensify in the inter-war period, but were very much based on beliefs about birth going back to 1900.

Conclusion

The 1902 Midwives Act, which was passed after bitter and prolonged debate, was very much an idea whose time had come. It chimed with ideas about social responsibility and concerns about the health of the nation, viewed through the lens of infant welfare in particular. Although it has been characterised as leading to the development of midwifery as a profession, rather than as a local neighbourhood craft, the evidence for this period suggests that this interpretation is rather exaggerated. It was, very slowly, becoming more acceptable for middle-class women to become midwives, and they were certainly over-represented in professional groups such as the Midwives Institute. However, the majority of midwives lived and worked in their local communities, earning low wages for sporadic work. Training continued to be the exception rather than the norm, and the most significant feature of the Act was the impetus it leant to the rehabilitation of the image of the midwife from dangerous 'Gamp' to potential propagandist for new doctrines of public health and medical hegemony, and the regulation of the lives of mothers.

The majority of women continued to be delivered by midwives in their own homes, although richer women favoured doctor-led deliveries even if in practice it was the midwife, trained or handywoman, who caught the baby. 'Risk' was not a word used during this period, and although there was an increasing emphasis on safeguarding the health of the infant, childbirth was seen as carrying attendant dangers for women of all social classes which could be faced down bravely but could not be ameliorated. As infant welfare schemes continued to develop in the inter-war period and infant mortality continued to decline, stubborn rates of maternal death would come to take centre stage. The next chapter will explore the longer term impact of midwifery regulation and education, as well as the political and scientific turmoil caused by high maternal mortality, and underlying all of this, the impact that the demands of women themselves had on changing patterns of care.

3   1915–39

Introduction

For pregnant women in 1930 childbirth was as much a time of potentially fatal risk as it had been at the turn of the century, and in some areas of the country the danger was actually greater. The maternal mortality rate (maternal deaths per thousand births [MMR]) was as high in 1934 as it had been 50 years previously, and maternal morbidity, although impossible to quantify, appears from anecdotal evidence to have been very widespread. The situation was considered to be particularly acute in some rural and urban areas which experienced rising levels of MMR during the 1920s and early 1930s. The first part of this chapter will explore the progress of MMR, its possible causes, attempts to tackle it, and its wider significance to maternity care.

The second part of the chapter will focus on the social construct of childbirth, and in particular the development of salaried midwifery and specialist hospital services. In contrast to some feminist writers who have argued that women began to lose control over childbirth in this period and the coerced move to hospital for birth and the development of a professional midwifery service, the evidence from a range of local studies suggests that the growth of maternity hospitals and homes was in many respects demand led. Additionally the 1936 Midwives Act, with its emphasis on support for district midwives, allowed for the maintenance of a significant proportion of home births up until the Second World War.

In many respects, development of maternity services in the inter-war period demonstrated the most comprehensive move by local government into maternal health and welfare. By the mid-1930s services in some areas covered antenatal, intra-partum and postnatal care, with the provision of council midwives, clinics and hospital beds. This appears partly to have been the result of the ad hoc extension of infant welfare measures, and partly in response to perceived failures in maternity care, with MMR failing to respond to targeted approaches. There generally appears to have been a consensus across political parties, and others including professional and women's groups, that alternative strategies such as the provision of nutrition were not relevant, and that only comprehensive maternity services would eventually solve the problem. Despite a swathe of national reports, responses on the ground were based along pragmatic lines according to what was considered to be practical and affordable.

Maternal mortality

Maternal mortality was not generally considered to be a problem until after the First World War, because it was believed to be at acceptable levels. In 1909 a Report by the Local Government Board (LGB) which considered the working of the 1902 Midwives Act confidently asserted that, as a result of the Act, deaths associated with childbirth were falling (rates had fallen from 4.81 per 1,000 live births in 1900 to 3.70 in 1909: Mugford and Macfarlane 2000: 598). As Chapter 2 has demonstrated, infant deaths had been a concern of local and national authorities since the beginning of the century, but maternal deaths were not initially seen as an issue requiring concerted action. However, as general death rates began to fall, followed by infant mortality rates, and more significantly as the birth rate continued to decline, deaths in childbirth took on a new resonance. Nevertheless, the LGB was optimistic about the future; the Midwives Act of 1902 seemed to be having a positive impact on maternal death rates, even though its effects were being felt only slowly in different parts of the country. It appeared on the surface at least to be a simple issue of cause and effect; put into place a mechanism for training and professionalising previously dangerous and ignorant midwives, and maternity would become safer. Five years later, however, the picture did not seem so simple or so hopeful. Although infant mortality continued to fall after the First World War even in the difficult economic and social conditions of the Depression, deaths in childbirth remained at best static and in some areas of the country had even begun to rise again. Successive government reports looked in vain for patterns and trends, but unlike infant deaths which had mainly occurred in poor insanitary districts in hot summers, maternal mortality was messy and scattered, with clusters of deaths in areas which seemed to have no common or distinguishing features. Rates reached a national high of 4.60 per 1,000 live births in 1934, with figures for some parts of the country being over 6.00. Despite, rather than because of, official hand-wringing, the maternal death rate began to drop sharply from the mid-1930s, continuing its fall off into the war years and beyond. The rate fell from 4.60 per 1,000 live births in 1934 to 2.93 in 1939, the main component being a dramatic decline in puerperal fever deaths (Mugford and Macfarlane 2000: 600). But the rise and fall of the maternal death rate had significance beyond numbers. Fears and beliefs about maternal death, and indeed maternal survival, can be seen in national and individual decisions made about place of birth and provision of carer, and in the exponential growth in ante- and postnatal surveillance during the period and in the increasingly bitter struggle between GPs and obstetricians. The language of risk and the belief in its identification and reduction entered the language of maternity care for the first time. Fox (1991) argued that maternal mortality in the inter-war period has always been an historical problem rather than a contemporary one. However, this seems to be an over-simplification, as both government reports and women's memories testify. Furthermore, memories of death in childbirth continued to exert a pull on official policy and individual action long after the spectre was seen to be largely vanquished.

Efforts to tackle maternal mortality were superficially easier to implement than those of infant mortality had been because the Rubicon of State intervention had been crossed with the creation of infant welfare clinics. Schemes to deal with MMR followed many of the same routes and utilised the same structures, particularly the expansion of Maternal and Child Welfare Centres (MCWC), to provide antenatal and postnatal care for women. However, the essential difference between efforts to tackle infant mortality and those to tackle maternal mortality was that, generally speaking, the latter did not work. MMR did not start to fall in response to state and voluntary action, and in some areas it continued to rise, peaking in the late 1920s and early 1930s. It was not until the mid-1930s that MMR began its sudden and steep decline. Earlier efforts, including antiseptic and aseptic regimes, midwifery regulation and antenatal care, exerted little, if any, downward pressure on MMR.

A whole series of investigations into the problem were undertaken by the Ministry of Health; Webster (1982) suggested that the sheer number proved that they were not calming public fears. None of the reports addressed issues of poverty and poor nutrition, even though the highest rates of maternal mortality were found in areas of highest unemployment and deprivation. The Ministry preferred to see the problem as one of inadequate medical attendance rather than economic factors. Discussion of the failings of birth attendants was increasingly focused on GPs, rather than on midwives as it would have been before the 1902 Midwives Act and their subsequent official rehabilitation. The medical profession was increasingly polarised, with GPs feeling that they were being castigated in professional journals and in the Press for carrying fever and for over-enthusiastic intervention with instruments. Some specialist obstetricians were openly beginning to call for the total eradication of home births, and the removal of all GP involvement, as the solution to MMR. Fox (1991), in arguing that deaths in childbirth were not the public scandal that some historians have assumed them to be, suggested rather that the series of official and quasi-official reports produced in the late 1920s and early 1930s made it appear that maternal mortality was an issue of national crisis, but that in fact, certain professional groups were using the problem as a way to promulgate their own views on maternity care. It is certainly true that arguments over professional hegemony between general practitioners and obstetricians were in full flow during this period, and hospitals increasingly mooted as a way to safe, modern childbirth, but issues of wider health and nutrition also came to the fore. Maternal health was not just about narrow sectional interest but was increasingly seen as a barometer for the health of society as a whole, just as infant mortality had been 20 years previously.

Hanson (2003) suggested that concern about maternal death in the inter-war period was fuelled not by concerns for mothers, but by the determination to protect the health of the foetus. Her argument was drawn from her reading of popular contemporary novels which she claimed illustrated the growing importance of belief in a eugenic master race. In reality, however, national concern about maternal mortality was much more diffuse and humanistic, with particular interest in the foetus not developing until the 1960s. Undoubtedly there were doctors trying to make a case for their way of practising, just as some mothers used arguments around the dangers of childbirth to demand hospital births. Scientists, politicians, health reformers and feminists all got drawn into the debate which was a matter of national, but also of individual, concern.

Women very rarely died in childbirth; more commonly there were antenatal problems such as toxaemia or haemorrhage, and postnatal conditions such as sepsis and, again, haemorrhage. These three groups accounted for the majority of maternal deaths.

Toxaemia, or eclampsia, was responsible for 15–20 per cent of maternal deaths. Attempts to reduce its mortality centred around prevention rather than treatment; many antenatal procedures which developed in the period, such as urine testing and blood pressure monitoring, were designed explicitly to diagnose pre-eclampsia. One case from a municipal hospital illustrates its course:

> One woman had attended the Ante-Natal Clinic regularly but became ill soon after one visit and did not report her illness until a fortnight later, when in response to a telephone message the ambulance was sent for her. She then had very pronounced toxaemia and was in a comatose condition. In spite of vigorous treatment she did not improve. She delivered herself of a still born macerated foetus spontaneously, but did not recover consciousness and died 8 days after admission.
>
> (*MoH Report Sheffield* 1933: 90)

Ante- or post-partum haemorrhage was responsible for 15–20 per cent of deaths. Another case report, from the same hospital, demonstrates its features:

> Another emergency patient was admitted in a state of profound collapse after ante-partum haemorrhage. The child was dead. After blood transfusion Craniotomy was performed and a hydrocephalic foetus removed without difficulty. In spite of all stimulation she did not recover and died the following day.
>
> (*MoH Report Sheffield* 1933: 90)

However, of the three main conditions, it was puerperal fever which fascinated and frightened doctors and patients alike, as it struck women who had apparently survived childbirth unscathed, and its repeated incidence could destroy the reputation of a doctor. It accounted for between 33 and 50 per cent of maternal mortality (LGB 1917). The condition had been effectively described as a contagious disease in the mid-nineteenth century, spread by staff, family or self-infection by patients themselves (Loudon 1995). Yet the deaths from fever only began to decline in the mid-1930s when sulphonamide treatment was introduced. Before this point once infection was introduced there was little that could be done:

> One emergency case was admitted with obstructed forceps delivery having failed before admission. She was then infected and had a pure growth of *Streptococcus haemolyticus* in her blood taken soon after admission. The patient was delivered after Craniotomy but did not recover from her Septicaemia.
>
> (*MoH Report Sheffield* 1932: 98)

The hospital was careful to point out that they did not infect her but that she carried the bacteria before admission, the implication being that it was a forceps-happy GP who had caused the problem.

The question as to why MMR was the last major mortality group in the population to fall, and the reasons behind its precipitous decline, is not simple to answer. This is partly due to the multi-causality of the problem, and to the difficulty of assessing the relative merits of the various solutions attempted. Difficulties of interpretation are compounded by the incomplete nature of the evidence. There were several problems associated with the evidence for maternal mortality. The first is that MMR, and in particular the important fever component, were notoriously under reported, with deaths often being ascribed to more 'acceptable' causes, as maternal deaths were unpleasant for the family and professionally damaging for the attendant (Pantin 1996). In this respect it was easier for doctors to cover up than midwives as the former were responsible for writing death certificates, and could ascribe a 'better' cause of death such as heart failure for which no particular blame could be attached (Ministry of Health 1937: 33). Although the notification of cases of puerperal fever was compulsory after 1893, rates of notification were notoriously low. It was suggested by some doctors that this would remain the case as long as blame for the condition attached to the medical attendant (Berkeley 1926). It could ruin a doctor's career if he was found to be spreading fever, so, as the LGB noted in a report of 1917, deaths from puerperal fever were, in some areas, higher than notifications, suggesting a certain 'laxity' in reporting on the part of doctors.

The second major area of concern was the possible impact of deaths by illegal abortion on total MMR figures. Contemporaries and historians have debated the level of abortions at the time, and how far they were responsible for skewing upwards the MMR by exaggerating the levels of puerperal fever, as the two components were not counted separately (Ministry of Health 1937; Ministry of Health 1939; Shorter 1983; Loudon 1986; Fox 1991). The evidence suggests that in some areas sepsis as a result of abortion was a significant proportion of MMR, but in other areas, 'accidents' of childbirth such as haemorrhage were more prevalent (Loudon 1992; McIntosh 2000).

The final factor which confuses any discussion of MMR is the introduction in 1936/7 of red prontosil, the first of the sulphonamide drugs aimed at tackling sepsis. It was discovered in Germany in 1935, and taken up enthusiastically in Britain in the following year (Colebrook and Kenny 1936). It appears that the drug had an immediate effect on MMR, which was sustained after the Second World War with the introduction of blood transfusions and penicillin. However, its success obscured two important issues. The first was that contemporaries noted that MMR was falling before the 1937 introduction of sulphonamide, possibly due to a sudden, and natural, decrease in the virulence of the infective *Streptococci* (Webb and Weston-Edwards 1951; Colebrook 1956). However, as Loudon (1992) commented, such natural factors had probably impacted on puerperal fever death rates for centuries; it was only after 1937 that historically low, and sustained, levels were seen. The second issue that was obscured by the success of sulphonamides was that until their discovery, doctors and researchers had very little idea about how to tackle MMR. This was particularly evident in relation to sepsis, with a constant stream of articles in the medical press attempting to describe and proscribe its spread (Colebrook 1926; Young 1928; Oxley 1934). Debate centred around the possible source, endogenous or exogenous, with strict sepsis and calls to lower the intervention rates the best that could be achieved (Paine 1931; Garland Collins 1934; Miller Wood and Camps 1937). By curing sepsis, prontosil saved lives but it did nothing to prevent its initial occurrence. In fact it made hospital deliveries and increasing intervention more acceptable because it removed much of the risk of death from infection.

The first national report on the problem of maternal deaths was published by the Local Government Board in 1914 and followed reports looking at infant and child health. The report argued that puerperal fever – which as we have seen was the single major cause of maternal death – could be vanquished if skilled attendance at and after birth was available (LGB 1914–16: 26). In this respect the report harked back to the intentions of the Midwives Act in putting the emphasis on care rather than the wider social issues which lead to much infant death. However, as the report noted, the picture was more complex than first appeared. In London, it noted, the death rate around birth was 64 per cent lower than elsewhere in the country (LGB 1914–16: 31). For puerperal fever, however, the rate was the same. If 'skilled attendance', which it was generally agreed was more readily available in London, could have an impact on risks such as haemorrhage, why did not the same appear to be true of puerperal fever? As the report continued, the anomalies piled up. Maternal mortality was exceptionally high in some rural areas, such as the counties of Cumberland and Cornwall. However, it was equally high in industrial areas of the West Riding, such as Dewsbury. Yet a huge conurbation like Manchester, with pockets of extreme poverty, had a death rate half that of Dewsbury. Even more confusing was the fact that an area such as Huddersfield, where a lot of public health work had been done to bring down the infant mortality rate, the maternal death rate was noticeably high (Marland 1993). The problem was compounded by the fact that with infant mortality there was a clear link between cause and effect, particularly as regards sanitation and poverty. The poorest wards in an area had the highest infant mortality rates. For maternal mortality there was no such clear linkage, and possible causative factors such as illegitimacy, women's work and parity were explored and discarded as being the primary factor in areas with high rates. However, the Report was clear on one thing and its conclusion echoed down the following two decades: 'A large part of this mortality is unnecessary, even in the areas showing the most favourable mortality rates' (LGB 1914–16: 60).

Major government-sponsored reports on the problem followed in 1930, 1932 and 1937 and all picked up on the theme from the first Report. As the 1937 Report commented, however, as long as maternal mortality was seen to be 'preventable' the public would continue to demand to know why it was not being prevented. It highlighted the move in searching for causes, from the broad sweeps of the first reports, to the emphasis on individual cases and individual causes by the early 1930s. The development of antenatal care, of midwifery training and of greater use of antiseptics seemed to have made little difference. In a report of 1924, Campbell had argued somewhat plaintively that it was impossible to find patterns in maternal rates. Yet another report of 1932 (Campbell et al.) looked at the particular areas which seemed consistently to record higher rates of maternal mortality. However, despite it being obvious that these areas were either remote rural ones or northern industrial areas, there seemed to be no clear links to be drawn.

The developing speciality of obstetrics had, through its practitioners, plenty to say on the subject. As early as 1919 one consultant had argued that the only way to reduce maternal mortality was to ensure that 'labour, even normal labour should be considered as an operation'. This required a gowned and gloved obstetrician, working under sterile conditions with the patient in the lithotomy position, preferably restrained and anaesthetised (Bonney 1919). Consultant Miles Phillips (1935) commented optimistically that 'the midwife and the obstetrician of the future, working in co-operation will, it appears to me, conduct more and more and finally all deliveries in specially equipped institutions' (McIntosh 1997). However, these views were not accepted uncritically by GPs, midwives, women or indeed policy makers. It is tempting to see the conspiracy of male experts flowering during this period, as Oakley commented:

> The main change in the social and medical management of childbirth and reproductive care in industrialised cultures over the last century has been the transition from a structure of control located in a community of untrained women, to one based on a profession of formally trained men.
>
> (Oakley 1976: 18)

This smacks of over-arching plans and conspiracy theories, yet at the time there was no sense that there was one 'right' solution to the issue of maternal well-being. It was not simply about replacing women with men or hospital with home. As the 1937 Report into Maternal Mortality suggested, as equally culpable as ignorant midwives or dangerous GPs was the 'rush of modern life' including radios, traffic, and the 'sensationalism' of the popular press' (Ministry of Health 1937: 117). However, although there may not have been a concerted pro-hospital movement, there was definitely an anti-GP sentiment developing, with GPs increasingly seen as the perpetrators of many of the problems, just as midwives had been in the early years of the century.

To understand why this happened, it is worth looking in detail at who was dying in childbirth and what they were dying of. The original expectation was that it would be poor women who were dying in greatest numbers; they after all had the poorest nutritional status and housing and least access to skilled medical attention. Any medical aid they did receive cost money, and it was therefore beyond the pocket of many working-class women to pay for a doctor for their pregnancy and birth. Midwives remained the cheapest option. In many areas, however, the situation was more complex.

One of Loudon's main contentions, supported by nineteenth- and early twentieth-century writers, was that maternal death rates were very sensitive to factors around treatment at birth, but little influenced by environmental issues. He suggested that the quality of care given was the main indicator of maternal income. Issues such as the quality of housing, quality and quantity of diet, and the type of work engaged in by the mother appear to have been only marginally significant (Loudon 1992: 244). A GP and researcher, Geddes, had commented in 1926 that:

> The statistics procurable all tend to prove that neither the patient's *social position nor her hygienic surroundings* have much, if any, influence on her susceptibility to puerperal sepsis. Indeed it may be assumed that *the well-to-do in industrial districts* are more often the victims of puerperal sepsis than those in humbler circumstances. Therefore *poverty is not a factor* in the causation of puerperal fever.
>
> [italics in original] (Geddes 1926: 92–3)

Looking back on the period Winter argued that: 'To have demonstrated that the risks of puerperal sepsis as one went down the social scale was to show the impossibility of making a direct link between economic insecurity and maternal mortality' (Winter 1979: 455).

The 1937 Government Report into Maternal Mortality supported this contention, citing figures for 1930–32 which suggested that the two highest social classes were at greatest risk of death (Ministry of Health 1937: 111). Crawford, a doctor writing in *The Lancet* in 1932, suggested that the rate was highest amongst these women because they were most likely to be treated by GPs whose experience would have been limited and whose assistance tended toward the interventionist (Crawford 1932). The evidence of Cullingworth for London in 1898 and Fairbairn for Leeds in the 1920s suggested that maternal death rates were higher in well-off areas and were accepted as proof of the dangers of high GP delivery rates (Fairbairn 1931; Munro Kerr 1933: 14–15). For example in Leeds, in the years 1920–21, the death rate was nearly 6 per 1,000 maternities in middle-class areas, compared to 3 in working-class areas. However, in 1929 the Medical Officer of Health for Leeds commented that although two better-off wards had the highest maternal death rates in 1920–25, the next four highest were working-class wards. He was cautious about reading too much into middle-class mortality, arguing that:

> A considerable proportion of the cases of puerperal fever occur in the cottages of the working classes, many of which are small, poorly furnished, and ill-equipped for lying in purposes. The mother, for one reason or another, but generally as a result of over-work and excessive childbearing, is often physically unfit to bear the strain of pregnancy.
>
> (*Public Health* 1927 40: 210)

Fox (1991) argued that the effect of malnutrition on death rates was never studied effectively, partly due to the possible implications, financial and social, of discovering that it was a significant factor. As early as 1903 the forerunners of health visitors reporting on conditions in Sheffield commented that many of the women they met were ' … anaemic and ill looking, not withstanding their homes were clean' (MoH Sheffield 1903). Considering the impact of the industrial downturn and unemployment on the health of mothers, the local clinical medical officer chose to see it as a question of attitude rather than hunger or tiredness:

> Worry is far more harmful than poverty to an expectant mother. The latter one can help, but it is very difficult to treat a worried expectant mother successfully, as the pregnancy alters her mental outlook and magnifies her troubles enormously.
>
> (*MoH Report Sheffield* 1926: 105)

Discussion of the influence of 'malnutrition' on women's health and pregnancy outcomes was hampered by the fact that there was no nationally agreed standard of what it constituted. Furthermore, poor nutritional status over a long period of time could lead to chronic problems such as rickets (which could cause a contracted pelvis, making a normal birth difficult and potentially life threatening), and mitral stenosis and other heart problems. These in turn might be noted on a death certificate as the primary cause of death, with no recognition of the nutritional deficiencies which had led to such problems. There were sporadic attempts to address particular issues through diet; in Sheffield Vitamin A was given to a group of antenatal patients as prophylaxis against sepsis in the early 1930s. The results were inconclusive. Nationally Janet Campbell, the Medical Officer for Maternal and Child Health at the Ministry of Health, agreed that 'It is likely that nutrition plays a larger role in maternal morbidity than is generally realised.' (Campbell et al. 1932: 8). There was also the argument that moving out of slum areas with their shared toilets and outside taps actually caused more problems than they solved: 'when people moved from the slums, they bought new furniture on the hire purchase system, and this coupled with their rents and rates and transport expenses meant that in many cases they were going short of food.' (*Sheffield Telegraph* 2.10.1936).

Efforts to tackle maternal mortality were hampered by the fact that there was a multiplicity of causative factors, and that none of the schemes suggested for regulation or amelioration seemed to have any impact. Nevertheless the issue had a significant impact on the way that maternity care developed in the inter-war period.

Changing patterns of care

Concerns about maternal death combined with other developments in this period to result in new ideas and new language being used around maternity. These included the identification of the concept of risk, particularly in child-birth, and the growth of a motherhood 'industry'. This section will look at these developments, and will argue that they impacted on maternity care at several levels. Most clearly they led to the creation of ante- and postnatal care along the models of infant welfare created before the First World War. These were both designed explicitly with concepts of risk identification and surveil-lance at their heart. Added to this was the growing parade of books, articles and lectures aimed at giving advice to the pregnant woman as a way of sharing information about what was considered to be the best and safest behaviours, in order not only to reduce risk but to remind mothers of their sacred duty at a time when scare stories about maternal deaths might be making them think twice. Motherhood was seen as a matter of national sig-nificance, and regulation, whether through clinics or books of advice, helped to propel it from a private act to a public duty.

Researchers have often placed the concept of the development of risk in maternity care in the wider context of the medicalisation of pregnancy and birth. The very title of Oakley's 1984 book *The Captured Womb* illustrated her views on the development of antenatal care. The female, pregnant body was no longer to be the private preserve of mothers and midwives, but was to be laid open to medical surveillance and control. She argued that this idea developed quickly between 1915 and 1939 with the growth in antenatal care aimed at identifying, minimising and controlling risk in no particular order. Murphy-Lawless (1998) described the attractions and challenges of basing obstetric care on particular concepts of risk. In a reading more sophisticated than that of Oakley or Kitzinger (2006) Murphy-Lawless argued that male obstetricians were as much at the mercy of their own beliefs as were midwives or women. Obstetrics held out the promise of a 'cure' for maternal or infant death, arguing that com-pliance with the right treatment or the right regime would produce a favourable result. Within this philosophy, risk remained a tantalising and slippery concept.

In order to maximise her chances of survival the pregnant woman was expected to comply with care regimes laid down by doctors and the state. However, she was not to be a passive recipient of care, but in order to ensure success, was expected to look after herself to the highest standards. Books of advice on pregnancy and motherhood proliferated, although they are often overlooked by writers who stress that women were pushed to the side of their own pregnancies in this period.

In 1901 Dr John Ballantyne, who has been credited with first developing antenatal care, commented that despite progress, as he saw it, around birth, very little was still understood about the 'pathology of pregnancy' (Munro Kerr et al. 1954: 146). He believed initially that 'pro-maternity care' as he first called it would have a positive impact on the health of the child because clearly the only way to assess the well-being of the foetus was through the mother. It has been argued that his view reduced the pregnant woman to the status of vessel (Oakley 1984). However, Ballantyne had in mind not just medical surveillance, but broader ideas of support for women. He suggested that a 'pro-maternity hospital' would have beds not only for women whose present or previous pregnancies were indicative of problems, but also for 'more or less normal ambulant, working women for example who ought to rest during the last weeks of pregnancy but who are unable for financial reasons to do so ...' This was at a time when women's hospitals would still admit pregnant women with great reluctance only, although birth in hospital was gradually becoming more acceptable.

Antenatal care was further developed in the USA and Australia (Munro Kerr et al. 1954: 151–52) and in 1915 a municipal antenatal clinic was opened in Woolwich, south-east London (Marks 1996). By 1918 there were 120 clinics scattered around the country, both voluntary and municipal. In the same year, the Maternal and Child Welfare Act legitimatised this development by permitting local authorities to enact a whole range of antenatal measures including clinics, home visiting, dental treatment and educational classes. They were also allowed to provide free or reduced-cost food and milk to those judged to require it. Whatever the theoretical intentions around preserving infant life, the network of clinic visits and classes created meant that the health of the mother was also foregrounded.

As Marks observed for London, clinics proliferated dramatically with 96 antenatal clinics provided by the 28 metropolitan boroughs alone in 1932. Nationally there were reckoned to be 1,417 clinics by 1933, and this does not take into account all the ad hoc and voluntary arrangements which existed (McCleary 1935; Munro Kerr et al. 1954). Oakley (1984) and Kitzinger (2006) argued that the network of clinics increased the power of obstetricians because it made pregnancy both pathological and the preserve of the 'expert'. Murphy-Lawless (1998) agreed that this was possibly the intention, but it relied on doctors being able to achieve things through antenatal care which proved largely impossible. Just before his death in 1923, Ballantyne (Munro Kerr et al. 1954: 153) explained what he saw as the benefits of antenatal care.

They ranged from 'the removal of dread and anxiety from the minds of women' to 'the early and more satisfactory treatment of the dangerous complications of pregnancy such as toxaemia, syphilis etc'. Finally, he argued, still birth and maternal mortality would be reduced. This level of optimism about what could be achieved meant that when maternal mortality refused to fall in the inter-war years, antenatal care was one of the areas which came under scrutiny. Counter-intuitively, however, the various reports commissioned to study maternal mortality did not focus on the failure of antenatal care to achieve its optimistic claims. Instead policy makers such as Janet Campbell argued that antenatal care needed to be better organised and that more women should attend regular appointments. This is despite the fact that, as Munro Kerr admitted in the 1950s, it was very hard to prove that antenatal care had any impact on reducing deaths through pre-eclampsia, for example. One doctor, who looked critically at the results of the antenatal care provided by teaching hospitals in the early 1930s, found that although antenatal surveillance reduced the number of maternal deaths from obstructed labour, it increased the number of Caesareans and inductions, which themselves carried significant risk, particularly of infection. Post-war and current debates were prefigured by Browne's remark, supported by other research, that these operations were often unnecessary (Munro Kerr et al. 1954: 153).

Despite the misgivings of some researchers, antenatal care was very much a part of the policy landscape by the 1930s. The ideal arrangement was set out by the Ministry of Health in 1929, and its recommendations remained the basis for antenatal care until after the new millennium. These included the predication of 'difficult labour', the treatment of raised blood pressure and eclamptic problems, the investigation and treatment of infections and the education of mothers. In order to achieve all these aims, mothers were expected to attend regularly from 16 weeks of pregnancy. The regime of monthly clinic visits until 28 weeks, then fortnightly until 36 weeks and weekly until delivery was laid down at this time although there appears to have been no evidence base for this. At each visit the pregnant woman would have her blood pressure taken and urine analysed, as well as having her abdomen palpated and the foetal heart auscultated once it was possible to detect (usually possible after about 28 weeks, depending on the girth of the mother and the position of the baby). There was no indication of what action might be taken if an abnormal foetal heart was detected, or if palpation demonstrated an unexpectedly small or large baby. Original proponents of antenatal care had not seen the need for this level of routine medical supervision of pregnancy, being more interested in identifying pathological cases (Ballantyne 1914). The more detailed schemes developed in the 1920s suggest that antenatal care was perhaps being expanded as much for social reasons as medical ones.

It was made clear that women who received antenatal care were doing the best thing by themselves and their babies. As Oakley (1984) argued, it was a species of victim blaming to suggest that women who did not attend for care were deliberately putting themselves at risk. Powerful language was used by both the Ministry of Health and government reports looking at maternal mortality:

> The patient herself is often her own worst enemy, whether from ignorance or apathy, ill health or prejudice etc and until she is able and willing to co-operate doctors' and nurses' attempts to assist her can never be fully effective.
>
> (Ministry of Health 1930)

As he opened the new wing of Willesden maternity hospital in 1934 Sir Comyns Berkeley, consultant obstetric surgeon to the Middlesex Hospital in London, commented that the continued high rate of maternal death was caused by local authorities not offering antenatal care, and women not taking it up (*Manchester Guardian* 31.12.1934). However, the connection he made between antenatal care and well-being was decidedly over-optimistic. Records from the Jessop Hospital in Sheffield suggest that antenatal care was no guarantee of maternal survival, as Table 3.1 demonstrates. A researcher into the condition commented in 1926 that 'Antenatal supervision … will not affect 75% of the victims of puerperal sepsis'; a comment that seems to be borne out by the evidence (Geddes 1926).

Yet however dubious their success rate in terms of risk identification and reduction, women did attend antenatal clinics in ever increasing numbers. Clinics in Sheffield had been started before the First World War by both the Council and the Jessop Hospital for Women, partly in an attempt to anticipate problems in pregnancy but primarily focused on infant health, for example attempts to prevent still births. By 1933 the Health Department claimed that at least 50 per cent of expectant mothers in the City were seen at one of the clinics, and in Liverpool the figure was 74 per cent. Whatever their outcomes, antenatal clinics fulfilled a need: 'Now if there had been such a thing as a Maternity Centre where I could have sent for someone, or could

Table 3.1 Maternal deaths and antenatal care at the Jessop Hospital for Women, 1930–36

	Number of maternal deaths	*Received antenatal care*	*Did not receive antenatal care*	*Not stated*
1930	32	19	8	5
1931	21	14	5	2
1932	16	14	2	0
1933	16	13	1	2
1934	19	12	4	3
1935	19	12	0	7
1936	10	7	1	2

Source: Adapted from *Jessop Hospital for Women Annual Reports*
Note: Antenatal clinic attendance figures were not recorded before 1930

have attended without that feeling of expense, I could have been relieved of all that suffering' (Llewelyn Davies 1915: 34).

Interestingly in Sheffield over half the cases seen throughout this period attended clinic not on the advice of health professionals, but through the recommendations of friends. For example, in 1923, of 256 new cases seen in the clinics, 104 were advised by friends; and in 1927, of 1,281 new cases, 770 were advised by friends. Despite the ideas of some writers of a community of working-class women passing on advice and information about pregnancy and birth (Mitchell and Oakley 1976; Ehrenreich and English 1979; Oakley 1980), many women appear to have been very ignorant about all aspects of the experience (Humphries and Gordon 1993; Leap and Hunter 1993; Smith 1997). The fact that many took the advice of friends to attend clinics does suggest a common cause, however. Women appear to have been convinced of the need for more supervision and 'scientific' knowledge. This does point at reasons for the popularity of antenatal clinics, although as most women seem to have attended only once and as clinics were often over-crowded and inconvenient, it is uncertain what quality of assistance they would have received and how far it would have matched their needs.

For those women who did receive antenatal care the variety of place and type was huge. Women booked with doctors or midwives from 14 weeks of pregnancy to 35 weeks, and had care at local authority clinics, at hospital clinics, by midwives, GPs or obstetricians. Some booked doctors or midwives but received no antenatal care, some booked both and some booked neither even though they might be close to delivery. Equally interestingly, women who did receive care, and where problems such as raised blood pressure or oedema were noted, had very little in the way of treatment:

> 1st gravida, aet [age] 29, at 28th week. Under own doctor for ante-natal care. History of swollen feet and face throughout, with albuminuria. On 12th July labour began and her doctor was called. Three hours later she became unconscious and was admitted to Maternity Department [of the Jessop Hospital] … BP 170/110; still unconscious. Urine contained albumin ++. She died within an hour.
>
> (*Jessop Hospital Annual Report* 1933: 38)

Perhaps it is therefore not surprising that attendance by women was sometimes sporadic. Claims were made for the efficacy of antenatal care which were impossible to carry through. Marks explored the varied nature of care offered, with the regime insisted on by the Ministry of Health rarely being available (Marks 1996). Contemporary attention was drawn to this by the Departmental Committee on Maternal Mortality and Morbidity which reported in 1929 that 'There is too little antenatal supervision by general practitioners, and what there is is often too perfunctory to deserve the name.' This may have been partly because family doctors did not necessarily buy into an obstetric view of pregnancy care, but it was almost certainly exacerbated by the fact that general practitioners served growing clienteles and antenatal care was time consuming.

For midwives, who were also expected to offer antenatal services, surveillance was part of a developing relationship. A midwife who worked in the 1930s explained where she felt midwives stood in relation to GPs:

> I think a midwife, a good midwife, is every bit as good as a doctor because she is doing it all the time ... a lot of midwives were extremely clever in those days and you didn't have the all the aids that they have now. I mean they put something round a mother's tummy and they can see the heart beating whereas we, if we wanted to know the baby was alright and it wasn't getting distressed, you'd put a cloth on the mummy's tum and put your ear down to it and hear it that way.
>
> (Nottingham interview)

Another midwife, who worked during this period, explained how she operated:

> ... you used to watch hands, feet and eyes to see if there was any swelling. I used to visit them in their homes and if they offered me a cup of tea – even if tea was nearly coming out of my ears – I would have a cup so that I could watch the woman and get to know her because if you got to know the woman you could soon tell if there was any abnormality ... I was at their beck and call. I liked to feel I was a personal friend.
>
> (Smith 1997: 21)

Alice, who worked on the district in Blackpool in the 1930s, explained that she did not do any 'obstetric' work such as blood pressures, although she did palpate. Again it was the relationship that was central to antenatal care:

> Well, this was what happened. I was engaged as a midwife – straight away I went to see them and I gained their confidence and the trust in me, and I went every week during their pregnancy to see them in rotation, unless I was too busy and couldn't go but otherwise I went ... Yes, I went and saw them every ... I got really ... they got confident and they got the trust in me and they used to show me all the knitted things that they were making and we'd get really pally. I loved it.
>
> (interview Alice)

If there was a point to antenatal care, it was perhaps to do with this relationship, as much as surveillance. For women and midwives, it did not represent a brave new world, whatever obstetricians and policy makers may have hoped, and some writers have worried.

All the midwives quoted were working in largely working-class districts, and this may have influenced the way that they talked about the care they gave. For the middle classes, who still relied more on thinly stretched GPs than midwives for their care, there was a proliferation of books and articles giving advice on the best way to cope with pregnancy. There had always been a tradition of books of advice aimed specifically at married and child-bearing women. One of the most famous of these is Aristotle's *Masterpiece*, first published in the 1680s, and still available in Britain in the 1920s. This discussed all manner of sexual issues, including those relating to reproduction, in a manner that was always opinionated, and is believed to have had a wide circulation across the centuries (Fissell 2003). But the inter-war years saw the publication of books which arguably helped to change the landscape of reproduction in England: *Married Love* (1918) by Marie Stopes and *Natural Childbirth* (1933) by Grantly Dick-Read. Both books were aimed at, and read by, a predominantly, though not exclusively, middle-class audience. Between these two points, there was a growing body of works aimed at advising women during their pregnancy, and afterwards on the care of their infants (Hardyment 2007). One writer, a male obstetrician, summed up the need for such books of advice in the introduction to his own book: 'it is extraordinary, though none the less a fact, that Midwifery has throughout generations been surrounded by an impenetrable wall of mystery and fear' (Howatt 1922). A feature of the books was that they disparaged information available from any source other than a doctor: 'you will meet people who will tell you what a terrible time you are in for ... don't believe them – labour is a natural process and the doctor will help you and make it safe' (Birdwood 1932). Given that this advice was offered at a point when concern about maternal mortality was at its most acute, there is rather an element of hope in this statement.

It is hard to judge not only who read these books, but what information they took from their reading if any. As Mechling (1975) commented, it is important to be careful not to assume anything in particular of the readership of books of advice. Authors like Marie Stopes had a particular, and anti-establishment, view to propagate (1925). Others very much took the line that doctors knew best and that antenatal surveillance was to be encouraged, along with lots of rest, gentle exercise and the avoidance of any situation which may have been emotionally taxing; henceforth pregnancy was to be externally regulated. Respondents to both Smith (1997) and Leap and Hunter (1993) talked of a mixture of ignorance and knowledge, with information gained from magazines and books as well as from doctors or midwives. It seems likely that women took information from a variety of sources, sifting out what was useful and relevant to them.

In many ways, by starting with schemes for antenatal care, reformers, whether doctors, policy makers or authors, were tackling the easy portion of maternity. The onset of pregnancy was not always easy to judge, but it was time limited and had two concrete goals: the birth of a live child from a living mother. The question of postnatal care was, and has remained, far more problematic. To begin with it could go on forever, unlimited by time or investment. As contemporary evidence from Llewelyn Davies (1915) and Spring Rice (1939) demonstrated, many women dated long-term health problems from their experience of pregnancy and birth. Spring-Rice detailed the responses of working wives to a questionnaire sent out regarding their general health in 1939 and found that only a third of mothers felt able to describe themselves as being in good health, with an equal proportion describing their health as 'very grave'. There was, however, official reluctance to investigate the possible scope of the problem. George Newman, the Chief Medical Officer at the Ministry of Health in the 1930s, admitted that any official enquiry would result in ' … the demonstration of a great mass of sickness and impairment attributable to childbirth, which would create a demand for organised treatment by the state' (Webster 1982). At this point the government was unwilling to contemplate the organisation, finance or political will which this would entail. In 1936, Janet Campbell called for the establishment of national postnatal clinics, and called in particular for all women to undergo a medical examination six or eight weeks after birth (*Manchester Guardian* 21.3.1936). Although some Maternal and Child Welfare Clinics began tentatively to offer such a service, they were not developed with the same enthusiasm that antenatal care had been. Obstetricians, who were vocal in their calls for antenatal clinics and hospital birth, had no interest in the care of the mother or the baby after birth. For better or worse, therefore, those calling for postnatal care lacked an influential voice.

This is not to say, however, that no postnatal care existed during this period. Nothing was offered by doctors, but midwives, both trained and untrained, saw attendance during the lying-in period as part of their role (a ten-day period of visiting was laid down by the CMB). As one woman explained, 'The nurse came night and morning for a fortnight to check me and to bath the baby, and just mornings the week after that' (Smith 1997: 74). One of the traditional functions of a midwife had always been to wash baby and mother, and occasionally to care for them by cooking and cleaning for the rest of the family. Trained midwives did not handle domestic duties, but they did perform personal care:

> We had to swab them and to make the beds. Occasionally the mother would make the bed, but it was very rare. 'Nurse' was given 30 shillings to do this, she was getting paid! So yes, you swabbed them and then bathed the baby – that was for eight days – and on the tenth day you showed them how to bathe the baby and they could then do it themselves. But it was very hard work.
>
> (Leap and Hunter 1993: 179)

Midwives also acted as gate-keepers, policing visitors (Smith 1997: 74). Both mothers and midwives remembered trying to maximise the rest available to women, urging them to stay in bed for ten days if possible, and visiting them over an extended period of time if they felt maternal exhaustion or ill-health warranted it (Smith 1997; interview Alice).

A State maternity service?

The period between the two world wars was a time of flux for the maternity services. Debates around who should provide antenatal, intra-partum and postnatal care were a microcosm of larger debates about a role for the State in the health of the nation. Some writers have argued that women played a particular role in this discourse, partly by virtue of the fact that in countries such as Britain they had recently acquired the vote:

> Women focused on shaping one particular area of state policy: maternal and child welfare ... they transformed motherhood from women's primary *private* responsibility into *public* policy. During periods when state welfare structures and bureaucracies were still rudimentary and fluid, female reformers, individually and through organisations, exerted a powerful influence in defining the needs of mothers and children and designing institutions and programmes to address them.
>
> (Koven and Michel 1993: 2)

In contrast, it has been argued that most histories of the welfare states have downplayed the influence of women in shaping policy before 1939, and also their role as recipients of benefits and other aid. Work by feminists has contributed to this neglect by minimising the centrality of motherhood to the lives of women (Davin 1978). The reality probably lay between the two extremes of women as passive victims of welfare or as crusaders for change. Davin argued that 'The authority of state over individual, of professional over amateur, of science over tradition, of male over female, of ruling class over working class, were all involved in the redefining of motherhood in this period ... ' (1978: 15). Wilson (1977) suggested that the period saw the 'state organisation of domestic life'. This view represents what for some was an ideal, but was never a reality and over-estimated and over-simplified the role of the State. The inter-war period saw instead the development of what Lewis (1995) has described as the 'mixed economy of welfare', whereby there was no state takeover of welfare but a continued mix of provision by state and voluntary, public and private agencies. This is in contrast with the USA where a relatively weak central state structure allowed for considerable influence and autonomy by women in the shaping and implementation of policy. By contrast, France and Germany both had early and well-developed welfare programmes which left little room for the efforts of voluntary groups (Sklar 1990; Bock and Thane 1991; Fildes et al. 1992; Skocpol 1992).

One of the problems with the history of organised health care in Britain before the creation of the National Health Service in 1948 is the temptation to see all earlier developments as feeding organically into the implementation of the post-1945 system. Fraser, for example, argued that the welfare state was 'the end product of a very long historical process' (Fraser 2003). However, as Lewis and Webster argued, the centralised form which the NHS took was by no means a foregone conclusion even ten years previously, with the dominating theme, despite the creation of a Ministry of Health in 1919, being the continued existence of a multiplicity of agencies for the delivery of health care (Lewis 1986; Webster 1988). These agencies were capable of co-operating, but were often in competition for patients and resources. This was clearly true of midwives, GPs and obstetricians. It could also be seen with voluntary and Poor Law hospitals, charities and municipal services. It was argued, by Lord Dawson of Penn who led a review into the situation, that measures such as the Maternal and Child Welfare Act of 1918 contributed to a 'State medical service by instalments, almost by stealth' focused on local government. As well as the struggle between GPs and obstetricians, and between doctors and midwives for the control of childbirth, there now appeared to be a struggle developing between nascent municipal health services and everybody else. As early as 1917, the *British Medical Journal* was worrying about the total removal from general practice of the care of expectant mothers and babies and deploring the appointment of 'whole time medical officials'. It commented that:

> The wise advice of a doctor acquainted with the history of the family and familiar with the conditions of life in the district can do more to preserve child life than any amount of specialised advice given in centres, or the distribution of leaflets in tons.
>
> (*BMJ* 1917, i: 430–31)

The redoubtable Janet Campbell was quick to pour oil on troubled waters:

> A complete Maternity Service must have as its nucleus domiciliary midwifery by doctors or midwives in private practice, but this should be amplified and rounded off by facilities arranged and offered by the Local Authority and made available for all women requiring them.
>
> (Campbell 1927: 33)

She further insisted that 'By a complete Maternity Service I do not mean a municipal or State service.' Despite this, the British Medical Association – very much the voice of the general practitioner – continued to argue against the concentration of maternity services in particular hands, whether they were obstetric specialists or municipal doctors (*The Times* 02.12.1935).

Hospital birth

The most visible sign of changing practice in childbirth management over the last 100 years has been the move towards the use of hospitals for normal childbirth. This has been the case not only in England but in many other European countries and the USA. The exception has been the Netherlands which maintained low levels of institutional deliveries (Marland 1995). Feminist historians in particular have characterised this development as one of coercion with parturient women losing control over the place and pace of birth, and relinquishing traditional methods of female support within the community in favour of managed labours directed in hospital, often by male obstetricians. Writers such as Oakley argued that women were largely passive in this change, which occurred for reasons of professional rivalry, and the belief that hospitals were safer than homes (Oakley 1976). However, more recent evidence suggests that these generalisations overplay the importance of traditional birthing cultures and underplay the extent to which the hospitalisation of child-birth was demand led, with women themselves calling for more beds to be available. As Leap and Hunter discovered in their oral history of midwifery in the inter-war years, there was no 'treasure chest of forgotten skills' relating to midwives and birthing culture. Pregnant women themselves admitted ignor-ance, and fear: 'I were absolutely thick, thick as a plank. I didn't know where the baby was coming from, and all the nurse said was, "Oh, well it'll come from the same place it went in"' (Humphries and Gordon 1993: 35).

Although it is often assumed that the push for women to deliver in hospital occurred in the 1960s, it was an important avenue of debate and action in the 1920s and 1930s, with the percentage of births taking place in hospital rising from 23 per cent in 1923 to 35 per cent by 1937 (Stocks Report 1949: 18). Given the volume of print and vitriolic opinions generated by doctors particularly, in the medical and lay press, it is easy to overlook the views and influence of women themselves. Debates at not only the national level but also the local level were vital in shaping the move of childbirth into hospital. In fact it appears that in cities such as Sheffield, voluntary hospitals and local authorities were wrong footed by the levels of demand, which left them urgently expanding hospitals, and in Sheffield's case creating a free domiciliary midwifery service, to try to relieve the pressure on beds.

It was not only in England that these debates were occurring. In her study of Wisconsin, in the USA, Borst (1995) argued that support for doctors came from women themselves, including one midwife who engaged a doctor for the birth of her own child. Famously, as Leavitt (1984) explored, was the case of 'Twilight Sleep', where women championed a particular cause in the face of opposition from many doctors. Twilight Sleep (a mixture of scopolamine and morphine) was an analgesic which blocked the memory of birth and of any associated pain. It required the restraint and constant monitoring of the patient (for this is effectively what the labouring woman became), and there-fore meant a hospital delivery. The treatment does not appear to have been taken up so enthusiastically in Britain, but in the USA the issue was debated in popular women's magazines, and championed by the 'National Twilight Sleep Association'. All this activity appears to run counter to the arguments of Dye (1986–87), Oakley (1976, 1980) and others that women attempted to resist moves towards managed labour in favour of women-centred birth. However, as Pitcock and Clark (1992) commented: 'Significantly in the wake of the Twilight Sleep movement, women had assumed control of childbirth and had sought to move its setting from home to hospital.'

In many urban areas of England the demand by women for hospital beds outstripped supply from the beginning of the twentieth century, before issues of maternal mortality and 'fear' became significant factors. In some cases this may have been because some teaching hospitals had a tradition of offering in-patient births. As early as 1889 the Jessop Hospital in Sheffield had 119 hospital deliveries, out of a total of 570 maternity cases (the rest were delivered in their own homes). This compared with Manchester which had 86 in-patients out of a total of 868, and Oxford which had 163 in-patients compared to 3,098 delivering at home (LGB 1892: 136). Things changed quickly, however, in the early years of the twentieth century. At York Maternity Hospital there were 64 hospital deliveries in 1916, rising to 201 by 1919. The Medical Officer of Health at York attributed this 'unprecedented demand' to mothers 'who realised the value of the peacefulness and skilled attention of a maternity hospital'. Eleven per cent of births in Manchester occurred in hospital in 1924; by 1933 the figure was 40 per cent. By 1921 there were 21 municipal maternity hospitals dotted around the country, including Hull, Sunderland and Leicester. Other areas developed provision by supporting voluntary hospitals: Birmingham Corporation gave £2,000 a year, and Leeds covered half the cost of available beds (Smith 1921).

In Sheffield the Council made provision for extra beds across the city to cope with rising demand in the 1930s, but struggled because of financial pressures. A municipal domiciliary midwifery service was set up in 1932 in an attempt to keep women out of hospital, both for reasons of cost and a lack of beds. The scheme started four years before a national Midwives Act which required such action, although Sheffield was not the first area in the country to set up such a scheme. Bradford Council already directly employed 7 of the city's 69 midwives, and even Barnsley supported one. Schemes were limited to the economically needy but medically normal cases, in order to relieve pressure on hospital maternity beds.

In 1914 in England, the Women's Co-operative Guild had been calling for the provision of a trained midwife for every woman in labour; by 1918 this demand had been changed to a call for hospital beds and medical supervision for every woman (Lewis 1980). Doctors worried that debate about maternal mortality was making women more anxious:

> ... the question of maternal mortality has become the subject of widespread political discussion, receiving great publicity in the lay press. Maternal mortality is a scientific and administrative problem which deserves careful and scientific study, but in the experience of practising doctors, the publicity which it is receiving today is tending to terrify childbearing women and, in itself, a cause of increased maternal mortality.
> (British Medical Association 1935 quoted in *The Lancet*, ii: 211)

The *Sheffield Independent* newspaper reacted furiously to this report in an editorial which called maternal mortality 'a blot upon civilisation' (23.07.1935) that needed maximum publicity in order to deal with the situation. Other papers took the same line, despite the optimistic comment of one doctor that:

> I am sure we are beginning at the wrong end of the stick when we talk about maternal mortality; I prefer to talk about maternal health. We know that women do die sometimes, but childbearing is not a disease, in fact it should be a pleasure.
>
> (*Sheffield Independent* 12.11.1936)

Loudon (1992) argued that women's fear of pain and death in childbirth was not a significant factor informing their decisions, but women were certainly wary of the possibility of death or at least serious disability as a result of childbirth. Recalling her labour in 1937, one woman in London commented that 'I wanted to go to hospital because I knew if anything went wrong, everything was going to be right at the hospital. They're magicians. Everything is right there' (Marks 1995). Marks suggested that high rates of poverty and poor housing, together with an abundance of reputable teaching hospitals in London, made hospital a desirable alternative to home for many women. Economic issues were also a factor, with hospital being a cheaper option than a trained and certified midwife.

There appears to have been little tradition of women-led 'community birth' in England, and therefore labouring in an institution may have been an acceptable option. Many women who laboured at home did so in silence and in fear: 'You didn't make a row 'cos the kids was in the next bedroom, weren't they? You didn't want to frighten them to death. No, I never made no noise. I just used to hold meself. Grin and bear it' (Humphries and Gordon 1993: 15). Kathleen described giving birth at home in the early 1940s with a midwife who had forgotten to bring gas and air despite the fact that Kathleen had asked for it:

> I got to a point where I was really in agony, and I was screaming out. The nurse came over to me and she took up the pillow and she said, 'Would you mind putting this over your mouth when you scream, because the noise might upset your husband in the other room?'
>
> (Humphries and Gordon 1993: 40)

Lady Florence Bell, who studied working-class women in Middlesbrough before the First World War, suggested that women did not want pain relief when they were in labour because they were afraid of its effects (Bell 1907). Significantly she also commented that 'it is illegal to administer it without consent, sometimes refused by the husband'. This has a bearing on power structures within the family, demonstrating that perhaps childbirth was not an exclusively female concern. Possibly also, therefore, women felt they were more likely to get what they wanted in hospital. As Marks (1995) argued for London, however, it was equally likely to be for other domestic reasons; one of her respondents argued that she preferred to be alone in hospital where she could 'get on with it' without having to worry about her family. It was not necessarily a panacea, however, with some women describing the fear and loneliness of birth in an institution:

> You go in there, I don't think anybody went with me, no, just you in this room, it's just like a little gaol cell. A cell, and in there they take you first into the bath, shove you, push you, get into a bath. Strip, into a bath, strip, into this room, enema, shaving then, of course, you've got this thick nightgown split all up the back. And you're told to just get on this bed, well, it's a table, and you're on there while you're examined and they say how far you are on and it'll be another ten or twelve hours. And then they're gone.
>
> (Humphries and Gordon 1993: 35)

Despite this, the period saw a gradual incursion of hospital practice into birth. As we have seen this occurred for a variety of reasons. By 1937 35 per cent of all births in England took place in hospital, and the stage was set for further increases in the post-war period as all treatment became free, and hospitals became the only places to guarantee certain types of care such as pain relief.

Midwives

Whatever the debates about the causes of maternal death or the place of birth in the inter-war period, the main carers of women in childbirth were still midwives; they delivered approximately 60 per cent of all babies (*BMJ* 1935: 364). The type of midwife who was working (and at this point she was always a woman) and the kind of work she was doing was beginning to change, however. It was given added impetus by the passing in 1936 of a new Midwives Act which created a nationally mediated salaried midwifery service to cover the whole country. This Act had arguably had a much greater impact on how midwifery was conceived and practised than the 1902 Act which had said nothing about the remuneration of midwives or their conditions of work. Whether trained or untrained, midwives continued to be self-employed, which meant that they were paid on a case-by-case basis. One of Leap and Hunter's respondents described the impact which this had:

> The amount of deliveries you got was the amount of money you got. I was charging thirty shillings. I've always been paid, but sometimes by instalments, because people hadn't got a lot of money in the early 1930s. A lot of men were only working half a week, then half a week on the dole, so they had very little income and there was a lot of poverty.
>
> (Leap and Hunter 1993)

Some midwives were employed by hospitals or nursing associations, which might give them more certain pay and relief. In rural areas in particular these might be small charities, or larger affiliations such as the Queen Victoria Jubilee Nursing Association (Fox 1996). Midwives who worked in this way were often dual qualified and functioned as both district nurses and midwives in their areas, a position which was both responsible and lonely:

> The life of the nurse midwife in a small village is frequently one of self-denial ... she must visit her cases in all weathers and be prepared to be called at any hour of the day or night ... she must exercise some choice in her associates, and must observe a professional silence about the cases she is attending.
>
> (LGB 1917: 97)

Several further Acts of Parliament were passed before 1936 designed to tackle the issues thrown up by the 1902 Midwives Act. The National Insurance Act (1911) meant that families now received payment towards maternity costs. In practice, however, much of this was designed to go to doctors rather than attending midwives. If a doctor was called out, he was guaranteed his fee, a situation which did not apply to midwives who occasionally ended up paying for the attendance of the doctor if the family were too poor to do it themselves. This situation was finally rectified in 1918 with the Second Midwives Act which gave the local authority initial responsibility for paying fees to doctors (which they could then attempt to recover from families). In 1926 another attempt was made to restrict midwifery practice by uncertified practitioners – the long-lived handywomen – who could now be fined for attendance at childbirth unless they could prove that it was a dire emergency. The evidence suggests, however, that they continued to operate, and that doctors would often cover the cost of fines where they occurred. In 1928 it was remarked that 'there are 29 handywomen in Dewsbury and not one of them possesses a bottle of antiseptic' (Cassie 1929: 333). In Birmingham the following year there were believed to be about 100 handywomen still operating, mostly under the cover of doctors (Cassie 1929: 333). Data from Wakefield City Health Department showed that as late as 1930 there was still significant activity by handywomen in the area. A register kept by the Department between February 1930 and September 1936 detailed 87 cases, probably those which came to the notice of the child welfare clinic. In a study of these records Wilkes (1992) found that 25 different handywomen were recorded, 15 of whom appeared only once, perhaps as a result of genuine emergencies. Others, however, appeared persistently; a 'Mrs W' attended 21 births including twins, a premature birth and a still birth. Wilkes suggested that in some cases handywomen made repeated attempts to call doctors who refused to attend because they had not been booked.

Whatever the position of handywomen, it was clear throughout the period that the number of untrained, *bona fide*, midwives was gradually tailing off in favour of trained midwives, just as the 1902 Act had intended. In 1908 in Sheffield there were 65 *bona fide* midwives practising, compared to 25 trained

Table 3.2 Annual caseloads of midwives in the West Riding, 1916

		<10	*10–20*	*21–40*	*41–60*	*61–100*	*>100*
Trained	Independent	37	10	12	4	8	7
Trained	Employed	29	8	12	2	0	0
	Total	66	18	24	6	8	7
	Untrained	10	84	92	44	37	15

Source: Adapted from Bullough LA (1917) 'Midwifery service in the West Riding administrative area', *Public Health*, 31: 126–32

midwives. In 1936 the last two *bona fides* retired, leaving 65 trained midwives caring for the women of the city. Nationally 87 per cent of midwives were trained by 1925, 93 per cent in 1930 and 97 in 1935 (Heagerty 1990). These figures hid a wider problem, however, which was that midwifery did not provide a living wage for any of its practitioners, although *bona fides* actually carried larger caseloads than their trained counterparts, as Table 3.2 demonstrates.

In the mid-1930s the Midwives Institute took 100 cases annually as its definition of full-time midwifery practice, in which case few midwives, either trained or untrained, achieved this level of practice in 1916. Data for other areas bears out the impression that midwifery remained a largely part-time, low-income occupation. In 1933, of 110 practising midwives in Manchester, only 50 were solely dependent on midwifery for a living, and 18 of those lived with relations. The remaining 60 were all married, and of these 45 were definitely stated not to be in full-time practice. In 1935 the Midwives Institute conducted a survey into prevailing conditions of midwifery practice. Analysis of the results for Yorkshire, Durham, Hampshire and part of Lancashire showed that married midwives vastly out-numbered widowed or single practitioners, and that 10 per cent of those practising were over 60 years old. Half of the midwives in independent practice surveyed had fewer than 50 cases a year; only 20 per cent had more than 100. A third of midwives earned less than £50 a year; one in seven received more than £200. The Report noted that 'except for a small minority, the practice of the independent midwife does not afford a living wage' (*The Lancet* 1935, i: 937). In 1911 83 per cent of midwives were married or widowed, and 70 per cent were over 45 years old. Twenty years later just over half were married or widowed, and just under half were over 45 years old. The profile of midwives was gradually changing, but midwives remained divided by age, training, level of practice and income.

Difficult conditions of service and uncertain remuneration were among the reasons why midwifery struggled to attract the better class of 'professional' young women that groups such as the Midwives Institute, and indeed the Ministry of Health wanted. It was also accepted to be arduous uncertain work, with no time off, and the necessity to provide everything from equipment to drugs. The 1936 Midwives Act was designed to address some of these issues, and in doing so laid the foundations of a 'National Maternity Service'

(Peretz 1990, 1992). The concept of such a service had been under debate since the First World War, particularly by the influential policy maker Dame Janet Campbell (1923, 1927). The Women's Co-operative Guild made the same call in its Annual Report of 1929, as did the Chairman of the Central Midwives Board (Williams 1997). The most insistent voice came from the influential members of the Joint Midwifery Council, whose work has been analysed by Williams (1997). The group grew out of the National Birthday Trust, whose influential members focused on the issue of maternal mortality. A salaried midwifery service was seen as being a cornerstone in the reduction of maternal mortality, as well as for the good of the midwife and her clientele. The Joint Midwifery Council produced a report calling for Local Authorities to provide and administer a municipal midwifery service. This would run alongside the work of independent midwives and would be based on a domiciliary pattern, demonstrating that despite the growth in institutional births over the period, nobody was suggesting that the hospital should be the default place of care and birth. Midwives would be salaried with pensions, and those midwives who were not joining the service were to be compensated for their loss of livelihood. The Midwives Act followed very closely the report of the Joint Midwifery Council; and acknowledged its debt. Local authorities, through voluntary organisations where appropriate, were required to provide full-time midwives for their area by the summer of 1937.

It is important not to underestimate the significance of the 1936 Midwives Act. In some ways, it was only replicating what many local areas were, as we have seen, already developing in a piecemeal way. However, it was much broader than that, not only in terms of midwifery but in terms of its wider social significance. For the first time midwives had pay that was not dependant on the number of births they attended; this was vital at a time of falling birth rates. They were provided with uniforms and equipment, sometimes even with housing as the new council estates developed. They were also the first of the professional groups where no marriage bar operated (unlike, for example, teaching where women had to give up work on marriage). Individual hospitals might not allow married women to train or to work, but it was accepted that not only were many skilled midwives also married women, but many childbearing women preferred a married midwife (Williams 1997). Beyond this blow for women's rights was the fact that the Act set a precedent in setting up a national health based service, based around the power of the local authority. It could be seen as truly the apogee of locally based state medicine. As far as labouring women were concerned, it also enshrined the home as the cornerstone of maternity care, a situation that did not persist long in England but has remained central to care in some European countries.

Despite the concept of a 'national' service, the scheme was locally mediated, and researchers such as Peretz (1992) have explored the impact of different local factors and arrangements (see also Rhodes 1999). Some of the differences were due to simple factors such as geography; midwives in rural areas had much further distances to cover than their urban counterparts, and antenatal clinics, doctor's services, and diagnostic laboratories were all used fairly infrequently (Fox 1993). Oakley (1986) and Heagerty (1997) both argued that the Act meant that state control of midwives had come in through the back door. Certainly there was a concern amongst some midwives that the Act would take with it their autonomy in terms of their freedom to practise (Williams 1997). This implies a level of organisation, power and concerted action that Local Authorities never possessed over the work of midwives.

That is not to say that the Act did not cause problems for midwives, and that some midwives did not feel that control was being exercised over them. Those who chose voluntarily to give up registration were compensated the equivalent of three years' pay, and those who were required to give up registration were compensated the equivalent of five years' pay. This did throw up some anomalies with so-called 'pin money' midwives, who worked to supplement their husband's wages, receiving the same level of redress as those employed full time (Munro Kerr et al. 1954). Moreover the bitterness between those who did, and did not, get employment could run deep as one midwife explained:

> The 1936 Act said that the local authorities had to provide midwives for the people in its area. Well, the posts were advertised and we all applied. In fact, it helped the local authorities to weed out the ones they didn't want. It gave them more control over us. Some midwives didn't get jobs and it caused a lot of hard feeling. There were four of us who had been practising independently in this area and I was one of the two who was chosen. One of the ones not chosen was a newly qualified SCM [State Certified Midwife] – she was a direct entrant [non-nurse] – and the other one had her SRN [State Registered Nurse] but she hadn't endeared herself to the authorities. She got a job the following year, but she never forgave me in all the time we worked together for getting the first job! She was a real thorn in my side. The re-organisation caused a lot of friction. Some of the ones that didn't get jobs took compensation – there was a scheme for that – but they didn't get much at all.
>
> (Leap and Hunter 1993: 55–56)

On the differences between women who were just trained midwives, and those who held a dual qualification as nurses as well, Oakley (1986) commented that the nurse-trained midwives were favoured in the reorganisation because they were seen to be more compliant with medical mores. This led her to argue that '... it [the 1936 Act] represented the beginning of the end of British midwifery as a profession concerned with the *normal* physiology of childbearing ...' (1986: 110). This view presupposes that midwives had anything which could be described as a professional status before 1936, which the evidence suggests that they did not. As the quotation above demonstrates, it was also not borne out by the situation in reality; nurse-trained midwives could be as difficult as their solely midwifery trained peers, regardless of whether they had an alternative view of practice.

Conclusion

The problems and policies surrounding maternal mortality and the wider issues of the development of the maternity services demonstrated the impact of pragmatic, piecemeal local authority led policies. Despite the beliefs of many feminist writers in the importance and durability of a shared, particularly working-class, female culture of birth, the evidence suggests that this has been over-stated. Practitioners and mothers were disunited and made little common cause. There appears to have been considerable demand for advice and assistance, with antenatal clinics proving popular with women. Over the hospitalisation of childbirth, women made demands for beds, drugs and expertise to which local authorities and hospitals had to respond. Women were not forced into particular patterns of care or to hospital deliveries through a lack of alternatives or the destruction of community-based patterns of care. There was considerable debate amongst all those involved in maternity about the best, and safest, way of delivering care, and the conclusions reached varied according to professional group, location and the state of the economy. Concepts of safety and risk began to develop, fuelled by the national scandal of maternal mortality. At the margins this did encourage a move to hospital births, but for women other factors such as the opportunity for rest, food and companionship were equally important. From a professional point of view, the 1936 Midwives Act signalled that midwives were now a respected, and respectable, part of the provision of maternity services. GPs, in contrast, were castigated during this period for their perceived responsibility for the majority of maternal deaths, and the specialist obstetrician and his generalist counterpart diverged with increasing bitterness over the conduct of maternity practice.

4   1940–60

Introduction

The period between 1940 and 1960 saw changes which impacted significantly the experience of maternity for women and for their care givers. The creation of the NHS in 1948 meant that women and families no longer had to pay up front for any medical care which they required. The right to a reasonable standard of health and of living was seen as sacrosanct during this period and made a huge difference to the quality of life experienced by many women. As far as maternity was concerned, the vast majority of women continued to be delivered by midwives, not just at home but increasingly in the hospital setting. Childbirth generally no longer carried the weighty fear of death or chronic ill-health, partly as a result of the NHS and partly as a result of the continued development of antibiotics and blood transfusions. As standards of living gradually began to rise in the 1950s, many women began to expect more from their experience of pregnancy and birth. Ante- and postnatal care burgeoned, leaving many midwives with huge caseloads and very little time off or relief from work. The period has been characterised as a high point for district midwifery in particular, with women cared for by midwives they knew and midwives having the satisfaction of providing the full range of maternity care to their women. However, the evidence suggests that the picture was more complex than this. Some midwives were overloaded and exhausted, recruitment and retention was a national problem and relationships with women and with other health professionals could be strained. As completed family size continued to fall, there was also a sense that some women at least wanted something different from their experience of maternity, and that it should be an end in itself, rather than just a necessary hurdle on the path to motherhood. This chapter will explore these different facets of belief and care in this period, and will consider the impact that they had on the central dyad of mother and midwife.

The National Health Service

At first glance it appears as though the defining point of this period is the creation in 1948 of the National Health Service, which, it has been argued, represented one of the most significant pieces of social legislation ever achieved in England. As we have seen in the inter-war period, maternity provision was the subject of much debate at national and local, amateur and professional level. Acts of Parliament such as the Local Government Act, which handed Poor Law hospitals to local authority control, and the 1936 Midwives Act, which created a salaried midwifery service, impacted significantly on the landscape of maternity care. Arguably, however, the inception of the NHS did little to change the structure or quality of maternity care provision in the first decade of its existence. Furthermore, neither midwives nor mothers recall its having an appreciable impact on their experiences of living and working with motherhood. The role of the midwife in 1960 was not dissimilar to that of her counterpart of 1940. Leap and Hunter (1993) suggested that for the midwives they interviewed, who worked from the war years into the 1950s, the 1936 Midwives Act was far more significant to them and their memories of their working lives than the NHS. For women, however, the minutiae of how midwives worked was of less importance than the fact that after the NHS all maternity care was now 'free'; there was no more saving for fees or hoping that the doctor was not needed. Davis (2011) has highlighted that despite the creation of the NHS being seen as hugely significant to the care of mothers and babies, the cost factor was the main aspect remembered by mothers.

Historians have suggested that the NHS grew out of the experiences of the Second World War, and the impetus which this period of national dislocation gave for wholesale social debate and change (Titmuss 1950; Leathard 1990). The seeds of such debate had actually been sown after the First World War when the Dawson Report (1920), under the auspices of the newly created Ministry of Health, suggested a unified national health service which would link preventative and curative services. The Dawson Report placed its stress on the provision of 'primary health centres', which would provide local services through GPs and the local authority and be backed by 'secondary health centres' staffed by medical experts. Although this model was not followed by the creators of the NHS, it did open the door to discussion about the possibilities of a national health service. Lewis (1980) has argued that the system which did develop piecemeal in the inter-war period owed little to any over-arching report, and more to pragmatic, local decision making. She also argued that it is misleading to see inter-war services as leading inevitably to the NHS, a view promulgated by historians such as Leathard (1990). The totality of the experience of war in the early 1940s – affecting everybody from every walk of life – is seen as having increased social equality. This, in turn, led to a belief in 'universalism' whereby all sections of society should benefit from the wealth and development of the nation (Fraser 2003). Addison (1975) argued that it was the twin experiences of rationing and evacuation which brought about this change in the national psyche. Rationing made everyone equal – and arguably increased the health of poorer families who now had greater access to healthy food. Evacuation made visible the hitherto hidden urban poor, particularly children, and made clear the effects of poverty and ill-health on whole swathes of the population.

Contemporary reports echoed and fostered this national sense that something must be done, and the emphasis on building a better nation continued whilst the War still raged. The Beveridge Report, published in 1942 and a wartime best seller, argued for the provision of comprehensive family allowances, a universal health service and the maintenance of full employment. Historians have debated all aspects of the Report, which suggested that the population of Britain needed freedom from squalor, want, idleness, ignorance and disease. It has been suggested that the plan looked back rather than forward, was unachievable, or alternatively that the principles it enshrined were unassailable (Glennerster 2007). The language of the Report carried through into the immediate post-war period and the planning of the future of Britain. In surveying everything from emigration to sexual knowledge among couples, the Royal Commission on Population, which reported in 1949, argued that everyone wanted, and deserved, a slice of the good life. These included women, whose reluctance to have large families was considered to have a deleterious effect on the future of the nation. The Commission noted that:

> ... it is clear that in general women today are not prepared to accept, as most women in Victorian times accepted, a married life of continuous preoccupation with housework and care of children, and that the more independent status and wider interests of women today, which are part of the ideals of the community as a whole, are not compatible with repeated and excessive childbearing.
>
> (Royal Commission on Population 1949: 148)

For the maternity service itself the NHS had two consequences, which both took time to reveal themselves and filter through. The first was that GPs were to be paid extra for providing maternity services, a fact which Towler and Bramall (1986) suggested led to a renewed interest in antenatal care by doctors. From the point of view of the district midwife, it also resulted in a diminution in continuity of care for women, as they would now go to their GP for antenatal care, but still see their midwife for the actual birth. Yet evidence from midwives working across the period does not suggest that they felt crowded out by the practice of GPs. In many ways the period after the foundation of the NHS represented the last hurrah of the GPs offering maternity services, for they themselves were increasingly sidelined by the third part of the NHS triumvirate of services, the hospitals. District midwives continued to be employed by local authorities, under the auspices of the Medical Officer of Health; a system identical to that set up after 1936. Their work represented one part of the NHS, with the services provided by GPs, often in small single-handed practices, the second part. These were both elements of a community-based service. The third element was based on the provision of acute services; in the case of maternity this was hospital-based obstetric services. The NHS took over the running of both local authority (previously Poor Law) and voluntary hospitals, and even though management boards were appointed, power lay largely in the hands of consultants. This was a deliberate ploy by Bevan, the minister who steered the NHS Bill to completion; he sought to negate the opposition of GPs to the NHS by buying the support of consultants through lucrative deals on power and remuneration (Willcocks 1967). As far as maternity was concerned, it led to a concentration of power and influence in the hands of consultant obstetricians who had a particular view about how maternity services should be provided. It also gave them a considerable influence on the development of government policy, particularly as regards the desirability of and provision for an ever increasing proportion of births to take place in hospital. The Royal Commission on Population demonstrated the extent to which the cult of the expert was developing even before the NHS was inaugurated:

> On the technical side [of maternity services] the main lines of advance suggested by expert inquiry are better obstetric practice, more intensive antenatal and post-natal care, the maintenance of a high state of nutrition, and the further education of women to make use of expert advice and help.
> (Royal Commission on Population 1949: 195)

One of the areas where perhaps the NHS did have a major impact on women's lives, was in the area of postnatal health. Spring Rice (1939) and others had drawn attention to the fact that many women lived their lives under the shadow of poor health for which they could not afford to seek treatment. National health insurance schemes had rarely covered women effectively, and when family resources were scarce the evidence suggests that women did not seek help for chronic conditions, which they often self-dated from their experiences of maternity. The NHS allowed women to gain treatment without up-front cost, and they appear to have used its services in droves; not having to scrimp and save for health care is what most women associated with the NHS in its early days (Leap and Hunter 1993; Devlin 1995).

The golden age of district midwifery?

The period between the creation of the NHS and the wholesale move of birth into the hospital setting in the mid-1960s, has been characterised as a golden age for district midwifery. Midwives were, through their training and practice, confident and competent professionals, who, whatever the rules said, were able to exercise a high degree of autonomy in their working lives. They provided the backbone of maternity care in England, and particularly in rural areas, were at the centre of community health care provision. Recently, as policy makers have sought solutions to the sometimes fragmented maternity care systems which have developed in the early twenty-first century, this period has been held up as an example of good midwifery practice. Rooted in their communities, midwives offered individualised family-based care. Furthermore, midwives working after 1936 were not dependent on the collection of fees for their remuneration; they were guaranteed salaries, pensions and equipment. The old debates about the safety and efficacy of midwives had largely died away after 1936, and they were seen as an essential element of a modern maternity service.

This section will explore some of these ideas and beliefs around the practice of district midwives between 1940 and 1960. It will consider the extent to which midwives actually felt they were working in a 'privileged' time and will look at some of the challenges of being immersed in community practice. Finally it will suggest that a sense of power and autonomy for midwives came perhaps at the expense of women in their care and was one of the factors leading to an increasingly vocal voice in maternity care: that of mothers themselves.

Midwives working in the 1940s and 1950s had all received some level of training. Descriptions of training in this period suggest that it was designed to develop a competent practical midwife as quickly as possible. Training had been altered in 1938 to provide two distinct 'parts'. The first, although including the delivery of ten babies, was primarily theoretical and hospital based, and was assessed by oral and written exams. The second part was largely or entirely domiciliary based and was designed to give the pupil midwife the chance to link theory to practice, and to demonstrate competence. Although direct entry training was not abandoned, the majority of midwives now came from nursing. This in itself caused problems because many nurses completed only Part One of their training; this opened up senior nursing posts to them, but did nothing for midwifery recruitment. Only those who went on to complete their Part Two were entitled to call themselves a 'State Certified Midwife'. One midwife, Margaret, who trained in Nottingham in the 1950s, described her route into the role, and her experience of the two parts of training:

INTERVIEWER: So did you always want to do midwifery?
MARGARET: No
INTERVIEWER: or just the chance was there?
MARGARET: I just followed on [from nurse training] didn't know what I wanted to do. And we did six months at the City and six months at the Firs [a maternity home], where three months of that time at the Firs you went out into the community. And I was on a bike, a pedal bike, ordinary bike and really enjoyed it. And so I applied for a job in the community and there was one in my area, in this area. So I went for an interview, I was offered the post before my exam results.

Another midwife, Brenda, also described midwifery as something you 'fell into' and commented that:

> I enjoyed my nursing career and then it was the done thing to go and do your midwifery. I was really only going to do midwifery because that's what you did, and I did it and then I got hooked on it really.
>
> (Brenda interview)

Midwives remembered having lectures from both obstetricians and Sister Tutors (now with their own training and qualifications), with a curriculum laid down by the CMB and supplemented with an increasing number of textbooks aimed purely at the pupil midwife (Johnstone 1949; two textbooks which continue to be produced today first appeared just before and during this period: Mayes in 1937 and Myles in 1953). The expectation was that students would cover not only normal labour and complications, but also ante- and postnatal care and, after 1955, aspects of mothercraft, nutrition and infant care and feeding. It was not, however, textbooks or lectures which were credited by midwives as developing their skills, but the practicalities of being on the wards or in people's homes:

> Well there were four of us from the general hospital, where I did my general training. We went down to Guy's to do midwifery, and because there were four of us, they put us on night duty for the first month. And so that meant I was put on the labour wards, but they were nothing like you have today. So I was thrown in the deep end, but the medical students were supposed to do all the deliveries and we'd be clearing up … At Guy's we were taught not to watch the clock and if they did breech, because in those days they did a lot of breeching coz they didn't turn them, they used … there was one consultant that always had the clock covered up. He'd say 'cover the clock up' to deliver a breech. So I always felt when I was on the district and I had a breech delivery, that I felt confident to deliver it.
>
> (Barbara interview)

Reflecting back on their training after long careers, midwives were proud and shocked at the extent to which they were left alone to manage their own cases. They described these situations as giving them confidence and resilience (Leap and Hunter 1993; Worth 2007).

> Then when you came on the district, you went with a midwife and then she would choose cases and say 'you go there and I'm there if you want me', which I always think it puts … Well it happened to me, I did it as well but you have to be sort of confident in your student really and she has to be confident in you, and then you delivered them alone.
>
> (Doris interview)

Once qualified, nearly half of all midwives were still employed in domiciliary work. This they usually did in pairs or small groups, sometimes even living together in order to provide cover for each other in times of sickness, holiday or to pick antenatal clinics and postnatal visits if the other had been up all night at a birth (Allison 1996). More and more midwives acquired cars across the period; sometimes provided by their employer, sometimes privately funded. They described the work they did and the impact they felt it had on the women they cared for. Doris described the hospital she worked in as being 'basic, but the patients, as I remember, were very happy. There were two Nightingale wards so you could see everybody and they were happy. They

chatted to one another and the staff. I think there was a really good atmosphere.'
They felt that this atmosphere carried through to the home:

> We used to do two visits [a day] for six days in the community ... if they
> had stitches we had to go for six days and swab them down. But if they
> hadn't then it was twice a day for three days, and then daily for ten days
> we looked after them.
>
> (Margaret interview)

The idea of caring was hugely important, as was the concept of camaraderie
and team work. These ideals did, however, bring their own tensions, particularly at a time of acute shortages in staff and a post-war rising birth rate. The
MoH in Nottingham commented in his report for 1946 that:

> The health of many midwives is being undermined by frequent night calls
> and overwork by day. It has been found necessary to take such measures
> as cutting down the number of visits paid during the puerperium to
> reserve the strength of midwives.
>
> (*MoH Report Nottingham* 1946: 44)

In order to examine this shortage, and the impact it was having, an enquiry
was set up in 1949 under the Chair Mary Stocks, the Principal of Westfield
College in the University of London. It provided a detailed picture of the
midwifery service just before the inauguration of the NHS, at a time when the
external status of the midwife was not in dispute, but the workload and
conditions of service were deterring many from taking up the work. The
Report noted how quickly perceptions of midwives' work changed; in 1929
there were 14,479 midwives to cover 654,172 births and the majority of midwives
were underemployed and struggling to make a living. In contrast, by 1945
with 2,000 extra midwives in employment it was proving impossible to provide
adequate care for 688,270 (Stocks Report 1949: v). Clearly the shortage was
relative; different areas had slightly differing birth rates and many midwives in
rural areas were also covering district nursing work. Beyond that, however, it
was an indication of how far the core role of the midwife had developed in the
1930s with an explosion in the provision of ante- and postnatal care, longer
visiting (up from 10 days postnatally to 14), and changing ideas about what
constituted a manageable workload. In 1929 an annual caseload of 100
women was considered reasonable. The Rushcliffe Committee, which had
reported in 1943, felt that 60 was an appropriate level and the RCM suggested
50. Despite this, over 50 per cent of district midwives had caseloads of 60–100
women, and a further 17 per cent cared for over 100 women. The Working Party
commented on the impact that high workloads, in both hospital and domiciliary
practice, were having on midwives: 'She is unable to give sufficient time and
attention to her mothers and babies, too busy to be calm, too pressed to enjoy her

work' (1949: 17). In domiciliary work in particular the limits to the midwife's role were set only by her 'physical endurance', a fact which contributed to the majority of midwives who trained never actually going into practice. The Report accepted that this problem was exacerbated by the fact that 96 per cent of pupils entering training were already nurses and often undertook training simply as a stepping stone to higher grade posts in nursing and overseas. This demonstrated how effectively nursing, which developed after midwifery (registration of nurses did not begin until 1919) had annexed the territory it wanted with midwifery increasingly viewed as a branch of nursing. The Report was scathing of this, arguing that it was not necessary or even desirable for midwives to have nurse training. However, with the training period lengthening, it did accept that it was hard for mature, married women, who were the usual candidates for non-nurse midwifery training, to afford the time or money to take up midwifery. This was despite the fact that non-nurse midwives were more likely to enter and remain in practice than their nurse-trained counterparts. In the end, however, the Report felt that however desirable non-nurse midwives were, direct entry training was probably unsustainable, and in the future all recruits should follow a core nursing curriculum, and take up midwifery post-registration (1949: 33). This was a recommendation that echoed down through the years, but was never actually taken up, although to all intents and purposes midwifery was a branch of nursing because the majority of midwives were nurses. One of the reasons it did not officially change was probably that although non-nurse midwives made up a tiny proportion of trainees, they constituted over a third of practising midwives, and without them the service would not operate.

The other side of the high workload noted by the Stocks Report was that in many ways midwives did have independence and autonomy that other working women, never mind non-working women, could only dream of. The Rushcliffe Report recommended raising pay to attract and retain midwives, and providing them with a uniform which, among other things, would 'contribute to the public standing of midwives'. Stocks agreed, arguing that recruitment and retention of midwives, at a time when there were a variety of careers opening up for girls, would be improved if midwives were regarded as on a par with other groups such as teachers, doctors or civil servants (1949: 26). Local authorities were required to provide furnished homes or other lodging for midwives, as well as laundry facilities, medical supplies and headed stationary. It is clear that midwives felt that such provision contributed to how the community saw them, and to how they saw themselves. In addition to these symbols of status, their workload was to a certain extent, controlled by midwives themselves. There was, however, a price to be paid for this. Increasingly district midwives gave their lives to their work. The midwife of the 1920s and 1930s was, in the main, married or widowed. Although there was never a marriage bar in midwifery, as there was in other professions including teaching and the civil service, the conditions of work operated as a de facto bar for many midwives; 56 per cent of district midwives and 77 per cent of hospital midwives were single

(Stocks Report 1949: 91). Leap and Hunter (1993) have detailed the extent to which some midwives felt regret over this, with one of their interviewees commenting: 'I often wish I'd had a baby ... yes ... but there it was ... I chose the profession.' This period represented the apogee of the idea of nursing and midwifery as a calling rather than as merely a job. For midwives working at this time debates over the professionalism or otherwise of the midwife in relation to general practitioners or obstetricians, for example, were often seen as irrelevant because midwifery was more than merely a profession; it was a whole life. The Stocks Report noted that the public and policy makers did tend to assume that both midwives and doctors gave up the right to an ordinary life in the pursuit of their profession (1949: 53). Midwives strove to provide a comprehensive service for 'their' women, and the continuity of care and of carer which was achieved during this period is one of the reasons why it has been described as the golden age of midwifery. The tensions between what women wanted and what midwives could offer were, however, already present: 'It is obvious that the patient's ideal is incompatible with any private life for the midwife and some concessions to practical realities must be made' (Stocks Report 1949: 54.)

In her work on district midwifery in Nottingham, Allison (1996) considered the impact that such issues had on the way that midwives worked. Although the recommended maximum caseload for a district midwife was 50–60 per year, Allison reported midwives delivering in excess of 200 women a year in the 1950s. This partly reflected birth rates and staff shortages, but was also an indication of midwives' pride in their work and the need for it; they would not give up 'their' women whatever impact it had on their workload. In order to provide this level of care, midwives had to be prepared to give their lives to their work. They also had to resort to other stratagems; one of Allison's interviewees, a retired district midwife, described how some of her colleagues resorted to drugs to keep going when they were ill or exhausted, or to help them switch off after months or years of broken sleep (1996: 13). Continuity of care, and of carer, was achieved, with Allison's research into midwifery registers suggesting that the majority of women were cared for in labour by the midwife who had attended them during their pregnancy. As a district midwife who worked in Sheffield in the 1940s explained: 'you never really got the feeling that baby was yours until you delivered it on the district' (Mathers and McIntosh 2000: 122).

One of the ways that midwives expressed their sense of profession was through their relations with doctors. The evidence suggests that there was a cordial and often symbiotic relationship between general practitioners and district midwives, although it was marred somewhat after the introduction of the NHS led to payments for doctors providing midwifery care. Up until this point doctors had frequently left the midwife and local authority clinic to dispense antenatal care and advice. After 1948, however, they sought to do so themselves. This caused tension with midwives who felt themselves deprived of the antenatal relationship while still being expected to provide intra-partum and postnatal care. Nevertheless, midwives characterised their relationships with doctors as good, and felt increasingly that it was a relationship in which they had a say and some measure of control, as well as a greater understanding of what women wanted and needed:

> And one GP, he was at the top of the hill, he used to like to come and give the girls chloroform for delivery. I mean at least he came out, but you got wise to this and sent for him too late. But he'd still get his fee for coming. But I mean the mums didn't want ... they want to be awake, even in those days they wanted to be with it for the delivery.
>
> (Margaret interview)

The same midwife felt that the relationship between her and the GPs she worked with was supportive. She described a baby which she tried to have admitted to hospital, only to find that the hospital refused to accept the referral because it did not come through a GP. In describing the incident, Margaret explained that the GP took her side and concluded that:

> ... the GPs did support you. We didn't get them out unnecessarily, but you knew they were there if you needed anything, and you really knew that you knew more about the situation than they did. But often it was the doctor who had to say ...

Another midwife remembered the midwives she worked for as a student in the 1940s and how they 'got on and told them [the doctors] what they wanted really. The doctors, to be fair, they would always come if you wanted them' (Doris interview). Part of this attitude was to do with professional confidence and belief:

> The doctor might come in but half the time they were observers, let's say to be kind, but you just got on with it really but one of those we had to send in because she was bleeding. She's still alive today and she's fine. So you delivered nearly everything, but it was recognising cases if you got them.
>
> (Doris interview)

In her study of midwifery knowledge and practice in the 1940s and 1950s, Rhodes (1999) drew attention to the pride midwives had in their responsibility for anything which they considered to be normal, and in their ability to recognise problems, and to summon help on their own terms. In operating in this way midwives were following the rules laid down by the CMB, but also asserting their belief in themselves as a group with specialist knowledge and expertise, who worked alongside, rather than beneath, GPs. Although not expected to deal with emergencies, midwives appear to have been more confident and pro-active in dealing with situations such as breech births or multiples than they had been in the pre-war and inter-war periods. This is reflected in textbooks as well as through the oral testimony of midwives. Johnstone (1949), in his textbook for midwives, described the delivery of a breech and for twins, with a doctor being called only for 'complicated' cases. Midwives described their pride in recognising malpresentations and malpositions which doctors had not noticed, as well as in delivering them (Rhodes 1999).

It was, however, in their relationships with women that midwives demonstrated most clearly not only their compassion and sense of duty, but also their power. It was the sense that midwives had of their own position and status which has perhaps given rise to the concept of this period as a golden age of midwifery. It could be argued, however, that this came at the expense of women and had a profound impact on relations between midwives and mothers. Some historians have suggested that it was the medicalisation of childbirth and the move to hospital births which eroded the centuries-old tradition of birth as a social event with midwives at its heart. But in this period, however much the State Certified Midwife prized her work and her community, she was distant from it. This was partly deliberate; her car, her uniform, her headed note-paper exemplified the distance created by training. She might not have expressed overt medicalisation, and indeed her work remained embedded in normality, but the status which she had assumed set her apart from her clientele. Even though she still lived locally, the midwife was no longer embedded in the social and cultural life of her community; she was no longer the woman who did, but someone set above and apart:

> As soon as the midwife's bike appeared, I sent the young one two doors up to fetch the cup and saucer. She was the only woman on the road with a matching cup and saucer ... we all borrowed it for visitors. I would run and wipe the lavvy seat ... I had four boys you see ... the old man would push his paper down his waistcoat and slip over the back fence to next door, he was really terrified of the midwife. I'd be left to face the music.
>
> (Allison 1996)

District midwives were conscious of this and used it to their advantage in a variety of situations. Doris remembered the two district midwives with whom she worked when she was a pupil:

> But a patient told me she [the midwife] when she was ill and she said 'You know, I'll never forget her because it was one Christmas and I was in labour and we had nothing for lunch and we were down on our uppers.' It was a family that had pulled themselves up. She said to me 'what have you got for your Christmas lunch then?' She said 'I haven't got anything Sister.' And she shared a flat with Sister Davies and she rang her up, 'Davies, bring that turkey over here, they need it more than we do' and she gave them a Christmas lunch.

Doris described the same midwife as criticising women's decor and the warmth of their houses, and explained it by commenting that 'She got away with it you see. They wouldn't today, but they were characters.' Being set apart had now become almost a badge of honour.

> But that was her and I couldn't understand – I didn't go with her much, she wasn't my midwife – why this patient said 'I've got Sister's tea.' I said 'Tea?' 'Oh yes, she only drinks Earl Grey' and then they said to me, another of her patients, 'I've got the enemas, I've got the Lux flakes and I thought am I supposed to do the washing? What are Lux flakes for?' 'I don't know' she said. So I said to Sister 'Got the Lux flakes, what are they for?' She said 'enemas, I don't use that other green soft soap stuff.' They all got it. My midwife wouldn't go to the back door. You know some farmhouses, they don't actually use the front door. 'I'm not the tradesman,' she said. They were quite bossy in some ways, but it was accepted.
>
> (Doris interview)

As Rhodes (1999) argued, midwives used this power to get women to comply, using language to reinforce their status; examples of this include describing women as 'good' or 'naughty'. From the point of view of the women themselves, these inequalities were recognised, if not 'accepted'. Davis (2011) detailed the negative impact that this relationship could have on women, although it was also clear that it could be positive and nurturing. As long as women were birthing at home they retained some control over their experience, because they chose when to call the midwife and how and where their baby would be born. District midwives were helped in enforcing the regulation of pregnancy by their own sense of importance and worth. The continued growth of hospital birth would, however, pose a threat to all aspects of this relationship.

GPs and maternity care

In 1940 district midwives were not the only people to offer maternity care. For general practitioners engaged in obstetric work developments in the maternity services during and after the Second World War exacerbated problems already evident in the 1930s. In 1937 the second government report focusing on maternal mortality suggested that only those GPs with particular interest in and experience of midwifery should be called to domiciliary emergencies (Ministry of Health 1937). The National Health Service codified this by encouraging interested GPs to join an 'obstetric list' and to allow themselves to be called by midwives when required. This list did not, however, prevent any GP from continuing to offer midwifery services. GPs were increasingly held to blame for past high maternal death rates, and were also faced with the growing self-confidence of others offering maternity services. The developing power of obstetricians and midwives can be measured by the Royal appellation granted to both the nascent College of Obstetricians and Gynaecologists (founded 1929) and the College of Midwives. GPs did not even achieve their own College until 1952. Some GPs observed in horror what they saw as the carve up of the maternity services between these two special-interest groups. As one leader in the *BMJ*, often the voice of the GP, commented: 'We seem indeed to be drifting into the absurd position in which the midwife is looked upon as the specialist in normal and the obstetrician as the specialist in abnormal midwifery' (1949). This was all very well, but had the danger of sidelining the GP who had always retained some involvement in maternity work, albeit with varying degrees of enthusiasm.

Evidence of the letters page of the *BMJ* demonstrates the landscape as GPs saw it, together with their sense of being blamed and marginalised on all sides as far as maternity was concerned. One correspondent described with feeling the cases attended by GPs, called to visit in an emergency when all the local authority clinic doctors who provided routine antenatal surveillance were long since off-duty:

> I thought of the good and bad sides of general-practice midwifery. If it goes well it is alright, but if it does not it can be frightful. All of you must have had similar experiences in general practice; the unexpected pre-sentations, the large breech in a small pelvis, the cases of inertia, the time factor, and even the simple forceps delivery that goes wrong. Perhaps you are just about to turn a simple posterior position. You have handed over the chloroform to the district nurse, when suddenly there is silence. You look at the other end, and there are the enormous pupils and the grey face. You drop everything and give artificial respiration. The patient starts breathing again, but you are now thoroughly frightened and hurriedly pull the baby out face to pubes. She's not really fit enough for a proper repair [to stitch up the perineum], so you put a couple of silkworm sutures 'right through everything'. Just as you think that all is well there is the dreaded sound like water dripping from a broken gutter. There is blood everywhere, on the floor, on the walls, and on your trousers, but somehow the patient survives.
>
> (James 1950)

Attending such cases could be uniquely stressful and uniquely exhausting. The majority of GP practices at this time were run single-handed or in small partnerships; the doctor who attended a case such as the one described above would have had to continue with their normal workload the following day. There were no attached nursing staff and often no receptionist. In the 1950s in particular there was a plethora of surveys exploring the work of the GP (Collings 1950; Hadfield 1953). They painted a picture of extensive patient lists with high levels of home visiting. Within this role, some GPs clearly relished midwifery work, others accepted it and yet others actively loathed it.

Some doctors undertook the bare minimum of surveillance laid down by the Ministry of Health, others saw their patients many times, although not frequently for normal labours which were still left to the midwife. This division made it difficult for doctors to make common cause in the face of threats to their maternity work.

Those who did seek to preserve a role for the GP in maternity often invoked the concept of the family doctor. This romantic ideal put doctors at the heart of family life, and gave them insight into the social and emotional status of their patients as well as an understanding of their physical health (Loudon 1986). GPs felt that this background gave them a privileged understanding of their maternity patients and their history which would not be shared by hospital-based obstetricians, who viewed people as cases rather than individuals. Midwifery itself, it was argued, helped to cement the role of the family doctor:

> Maternity practice is the very root of general practice; it produces the bond which unites the home with the family doctor, and the knowledge gained by the practitioner as family doctor not only compels him to see a maternity case in its true perspective but is one of the main guides in antenatal diagnosis ... to the obstetrical specialist the maternity patient is often little more than a case; he fails to realise that successful midwifery can be based only upon a co-operation between every factor which has for its ultimate aim the safety of mother and child. No clinic can take the place of a family doctor.
>
> (Logan and MacKenzie 1945)

Davis (2011) suggested that in the inter-war period GPs in rural areas particularly were generally regarded with great respect; not least because of the long relationships they had with families.

Interestingly, many arguing for the centrality of the GP in maternity work took the family doctor argument to what might be seen as its logical conclusion. Midwifery, it was argued, should occur at home with the GP at the centre of service planning. In making this argument GPs and their supporters suggested that domiciliary birth was not more dangerous than hospital birth, as some commentators were suggesting. Furthermore, they suggested that birth was not just a medical event, but a social one, and only at home could this concept reach its full expression:

> The new baby fits much better into the family when born at home, and no fears are aroused among other children that every time the mother goes away she may appear with another baby who will upset the cherished routine. I write, of course as a mere man, but I will never forget the thrill that even I felt when I found our daughter being nearly smothered within an hour of her arrival by her 2-year-old brother piling all his choicest toys on her cot as a present to her ... This may not be medicine but it is the

very stuff of happy family life and the foundation of a stable society. I pity all the fathers and mothers who are denied the joys of babies born at home and have to observe the strict and unnatural precautions that have to be taken in hospital if infant lives are not to be endangered by infection etc.

(Leak 1952)

Many women had positive memories of the care they received from GPs but the two-pronged attack on their work based on perceptions of safety and the growing hegemony of midwives and consultants meant that GPs struggled to make their voices heard. The seeds had been sown in the inter-war period with emphasis on the dangers of 'meddlesome midwifery' as practised by forceps-wielding GPs, seen as the root cause of much maternal mortality (Stacey 1931). In many ways the status of the general practitioner-obstetrician was, by the 1950s, analogous with that of the midwife before the First World War; GPs were viewed as a dangerous, ignorant anachronism without specialist training or knowledge in either normality or abnormality (Harvey 1950; Young 1950; Hadfield 1953). By 1959 a government report, led by the Earl of Cranbrook, exploring the state of the maternity in England and Wales commented that:

We have come to the conclusion that under present day conditions the practice of obstetrics requires the exercise of special skill beyond the normal competence of the general practitioner and a degree of experience that, with the present high institutional confinement rate, the average family doctor is unlikely to maintain.

(Cranbrook Report 1959: 7)

Apart from invoking the concept of birth as a social event rather than as a medical emergency, some GPs also sought to redefine domiciliary birth in terms of its perceived risk. If it was accepted that a proportion of births were safer in hospital then, with antenatal surveillance, it must also be possible to identify those which could safely occur at home (Cookson 1954; Salzmann 1955; Kennedy 1957). The language of risk and probability was invoked to argue that possibly multiple births and malpresentations should occur in hospital, but healthy women with uncomplicated pregnancies could easily be delivered at home. One researcher wrote of 'select[ing] cases for hospital delivery so that the remainder will consist of those who can be delivered at home in reasonable, if not absolute, safety' (Cookson 1954). Those selected for hospital delivery, argued Cookson, would include 'premature delivery, breech delivery and multiple births [which] carry a stillbirth or neonatal death rate too high to be acceptable for domiciliary delivery.' He felt, however, that there was no need for first births to take place in hospital.

Meanwhile RCOG had put forward ideas for a national maternity service, which largely did away with the midwifery work of the GP, in 1944. By the mid-1950s, therefore, GPs were very much fighting a rearguard action. The development of the NHS gave GPs some incentive to continue with maternity work by paying them for providing what amounted to a very limited service. It did, however, give consultants and teaching hospitals very significant power, and this was deployed against GP maternity practice. The Royal College of General Practitioners arguably arrived on the scene too late and its power was too diffuse to make a significant impact on the direction of the maternity services.

Reports and arguments

Although the work of GPs was sometimes characterised as dangerous and ignorant, maternity care in this period did not revolve only around concepts of safety. It was certainly recognised that the influence of sulphonamides and antibiotics, and the increased use of blood transfusions, did have an impact on falling maternal death rates. However, contemporaries accepted that these changes were due as much to generic medical developments as to specifically obstetric ones. The move of birth from home to hospital, which continued apace in this period, occurred for far more diffuse reasons than those concerned entirely with perceptions of danger and safety. Institutional confinement was mooted not simply as a strategy to reduce risk. It was seen partly in terms of offering rest to mothers, and partly as a way of ensuring the training of doctors and midwives. For many commentators, however, until the end of the period, hospital birth was seen as having been driven by wider social problems and by maternal demand at least as much as obstetric beliefs. Furthermore there was a perception, not just among GPs, that some of the reasons for the growth in hospital birth were transitory, and therefore rates would stabilise and possibly diminish contingent on improving social conditions. The Second World War had created wide social upheaval, with families displaced and separated and good-quality housing stock in short supply. Hospital delivery offered women a place of peace and safety, away from over-crowded accommodation and the dangers of air raids. The rising birth rate, and concomitant shortage of midwives, added to the argument for hospital birth, where there would at least be some level of available staff. In surveying the landscape in 1944, the Ministry of Health noted that 150,000 babies were born in emergency maternity homes over the year as a result of evacuation for one reason or another. It was commented that:

> The increase in institutional confinement was accelerated by war time conditions, including damage and incomplete repairs to houses, shortage of domestic help and absence of husbands and relatives on war service. It is too early to judge what proportion of the rise is temporary; but future plans are being considered on the assumption of a substantial increase in institutional births.

> (Ministry of Health Annual Report 1945)

Certainly for some women the experience was a positive one:

> As this was considered a danger area another mother and I were sent
> by taxi to Byfleet, Surrey, to a huge country house made into a maternity
> home for the war. It was 1940 and 14 of us arrived at the same time from
> Plymouth, Portsmouth and Chatham. Some of the ladies were very dirty
> because they'd been living in shelters. First we were bathed and had our
> hair washed with soft soap ... the staff were wonderful – midwives mostly
> who had retired but were called in for the purpose ... altogether it was a
> very happy time for me.

> (Smith 1997: 52)

The sense of companionship and support ran through this account and
many others, and may have fuelled the belief that hospitals could provide a
positive experience.

The provision of hospital beds, and the midwives to staff them, became
an ongoing problem. These issues were increasingly rehearsed into the
1950s as successive governments probed the reach and finances of the NHS.
The Guillebaud Committee (1955), set up by a Conservative government to
explore the money being spent by the NHS, suggested, very much in passing,
that the maternity services were 'in a state of some confusion'. This was as a
result, it was argued, of the continued tripartite system which meant that one
woman could receive care from a GP, a local authority clinic, a midwife and a
hospital, all in the same pregnancy. The maternity services were, as a result of
this remark, to be subject to their own enquiry under the Earl of Cranbrook.
This report was published in 1959 and although not signalling a complete break
with what had gone before, suggested the new direction that the maternity
services would take into the 1960s and the second full decade of the NHS.
Recent commentators have characterised the Report as the first in the triumvirate of official pronouncements (the others being the Peel Report and the
Short Report) which decimated choice for women, nearly destroyed the midwifery profession and promulgated the assumption that hospital birth was safer
than home birth. It must always be borne in mind, however, that government
reports tend to represent the ideal rather than necessarily the substance of what
was occurring on the ground, and this section will explore the Cranbrook
Report in these terms.

The justification for the Cranbrook Report came from the earlier Guillebaud
Report which commented succinctly on the issues and arguments as it
perceived them:

> Our witnesses have expressed varying views about the drawbacks of this
> divided responsibility and its effect on the efficiency of the service. Some
> have pointed out that the maternity services have been made to work
> smoothly in some areas by close co-operation between the authorities and
> officers concerned ... others have suggested that the services should be

brought under the undivided control either of the hospital authorities or the local health authorities.

(Cranbrook Report 1959: 4)

The Report pointed to a further confusion in the make-up of services that seemed to go deeper than bureaucracy:

The witnesses who favoured unified control of all the maternity services have pointed out that it would be possible by this means to secure a proper balance between the institutional and domiciliary confinements. There is disagreement, however, as to what should be a 'proper balance'. In 1952, the proportion of institutional confinements was 64.1 per cent, as compared with 58.4 per cent in 1949 ... We have been told that in some areas the proportion of institutional confinements may now exceed 80 per cent and yet in others it may not exceed 45 per cent. It is note-worthy that these figures do not necessarily reflect the quality of the housing or the needs of the patients in the areas served.

(Cranbrook Report 1959: 4)

The issues, therefore, were clearly complex and the Cranbrook Report can be justifiably criticised for an over-reliance on the pronouncements and pre-judices of an increasingly confident RCOG, which called for high levels of hospital deliveries. It is this aspect that has left commentators deriding the Report itself. However, a concentration on the demands of the RCOG means that other aspects of the Report are missed, in particular those which considered issues such as public health and psychological support for women. One of the areas that the Report considered was that of continuity of care: 'It is generally agreed that, ideally, one person in whom the mother has confidence should be responsible personally for both her ante-natal care and delivery ...' (1959: 16). The Report did note, however, that such care was hard to achieve in the hospital setting, and commented that relatives should not be excluded: 'In hospital her husband or a relation should be allowed to stay with her, if she wishes it, at least during the first stage of labour.'

In many respects, far from providing an official edict on place of birth, the Report was playing catch-up. Much has been made of the fact that it called for hospital beds to be made available for 70 per cent of births, but there was another narrative running through the Report, and that was that women were voting with their feet and booking hospitals for their births. This was causing pressure on the system, because there were not enough beds to accommodate all who wanted them, and all for whom the new ideas of risk suggested should be in hospital. According to the Report, some of its witnesses were quite clear that '... beds in maternity hospitals should certainly provided for medical and social cases but not to suit the conveniences or preferences of women who could safely be delivered at home ...' (1959: 18).

In the end the Report did not completely satisfy anyone; it agreed that more hospital beds should be provided, but argued also that for reasons of cost if nothing else an effective domiciliary service needed to be maintained. It did, however, cast light on one unforeseen consequence of a developing hospital service. Whilst women may have chosen to birth in hospitals, very few midwives wanted to work in them. There was a chronic shortage of hospital midwives, and this was accepted to be a significant obstacle to expanding hospital care and to providing continuity of care in labour. It was commented that 'We received evidence which indicated that domiciliary work attracted many midwives who would not in fact practise at all if they had to work in a hospital' (1959: 32). Furthermore midwives felt that they had a better relationship with women and families, and practised more autonomously than hospital midwives. This reinforces the concept of district midwives as professionally self-confident at this time.

Although the headline recommendations of the Cranbrook Report have resonated with historians, and the belief in the efficacy of hospital birth for dealing with issues much criticised, some of the detail of witness evidence demonstrates that there was not just one thread at this time. There were concerns expressed in several quarters about not just physical safety of birth but about its social and psychological dimensions. Concepts of choice, control and continuity of care for women were debated, and not dismissed (1959: 75). Women had agency, and to a certain extent the maternity services were constantly engaged in scrambling to meet the expectations of women.

These expectations can be demonstrated by the demand for hospital beds by women which, as in the inter-war period, tended to outstrip supply. In 1940 the MoH for Nottingham commented plaintively:

> The number of home confinements is falling as facilities for hospital midwifery increase, but there is a great deal to be said for confinement at home in normal cases now that home midwifery is so closely supervised. The use of maternity beds in the hospitals is now rather heavy and it may soon be necessary to insist that normal cases should remain at home where home conditions are good.
>
> (*MoH Report Nottingham* 1940: 20)

In 1944 the Ministry of Health noted that 'To meet the increased demand for institutional confinements, about 425 new maternity beds were provided during the year, and with difficulty both midwives and domestic staff were obtained' (Ministry of Health 1944: 23). Clearly these were beds provided for women at low obstetric risk as there was no mention of the need for more doctors; it was the social demands of maternity that the Ministry was trying to assuage. A steeply rising birth rate at the end of the war put the maternity services under even greater pressure, with the number of births in England and Wales 20,000 higher in the spring of 1946 than they had been the previous autumn (Ministry of Health 1947: 68). The Ministry became fixated on efforts to get women out of hospital earlier in the postnatal period, and anxiously charted every change in the figures. During the war women had often of necessity been ambulant very early, if only to get to bomb shelters. The idea that it was not dangerous but could be beneficial to be out of bed before the end of the first postnatal week gradually spread (Ministry of Health 1949: 158). It was still common practice, however, for women to remain in hospital for ten days, and the period showed only a gradual reduction in this despite the continued pressure on bed space. In 1955 the mean postnatal stay in hospital was 11 days; by 1959 this had dropped to 9.3 with nearly 20 per cent of women being discharged before 7 days (Ministry of Health 1963: 31). This allowed for some increase in numbers of women delivered in hospital even though the number of hospital beds remained static. Early ambulation was not considered by some to be particularly helpful. One textbook for midwives explained that:

> During her hospital training the pupil midwife will find that the normal patient is allowed out of bed on the seventh day or thereby, and discharged on the tenth day. This is by no means ideal, but conditions in most maternity hospitals are governed by two factors: (1) the reluctance of the patient to stay more than the minimal time in hospital because of worrying about her husband and her home, and (2) because keeping a healthy puerperal patient in hospital for longer than that period may prevent the admission of a new patient in labour.
>
> (Johnstone 1949: 159)

Johnstone went on to argue that all women should stay in bed for at least eight to ten days, and therefore rise only slowly. However, as in all areas of maternity, there were other voices calling for earlier rising, with 48 hours regarded as equally safe (Carter 1948).

Women themselves had mixed views on their hospital stays. Doris, whose son was born in 1938, commented that:

> Those were the days when we stayed in the maternity hospital for fourteen days. The old wives' tale was that if we put our feet on the floor under ten days we would drop down dead. That's the truth! So we came home after fourteen days, weak as water and never having seen the baby bathed.
>
> (Devlin 1995: 100)

Twenty years later Liz had a more positive experience of her stay: 'With the first baby I was in hospital for ten days. I'd never seen a newborn baby before – and they taught me how to bath it and got me going with breastfeeding ...' (Devlin 1995: 115).

By 1959 65 per cent of all births occurred in hospital, but this headline figure disguised many debates and variations, with place of birth being very much dependant on region. Only 47 per cent of women in East Anglia had a hospital birth, compared to 68.5 per cent in London. Some of this was due to necessity; East Anglia was a rural area with no large concentrations of population, and local midwives served as district nurses and sometimes health visitors as well as midwives, and were therefore very much embedded in their communities. A doctor who worked in the area during the Second World War described conditions:

> We would come to a fence, abandon the car, and clamber over the stile and across the fields in the pitch black. Eventually we would come to the house which would be very primitive and broken down. They had been good cottages but no repairs had been done and these families were very poor people ... some houses were appalling, with no plumbing and filthy unhygienic conditions ... If anything had gone wrong, heaven knows what we would have done. Ipswich was about twenty-five miles away, in the black-out, and there was no telephone for miles.
>
> (Devlin 1995: 105)

In London the problem was perceived to be huge and growing; there were not enough beds to accommodate all those who wanted to deliver in hospital. As early as 1945 it was noted that the proportion of hospital deliveries had risen from one-third to one-half of total births during the war. There was still, however, a significant level of unmet demand which had nothing to do with perceptions of risk. In 1959 87.2 per cent of women who had their babies in hospital had spontaneous deliveries, and there was a national forceps rate of 7.3 per cent and Caesarean section rate of 4.4 per cent. Just as significantly, over a quarter of women booked their hospital birth before the fourth month of pregnancy; for many women this was a planned move. In London this situation led to the ad hoc expansion of what were deemed 'emergency beds' to try and provide space for women who, at the last minute, needed a hospital birth for medical or social reasons. Many commentators expressed frustration that beds were being taken by women who did not 'need' them, while those considered high risk, such as grand multiparae, tended to deliver at home (Ministry of Health 1959: 158). Allison's (1996) work on Nottingham demonstrated that concepts of selection for hospital delivery on the basis of obstetric or social risk were very hit-and-miss. Some women were refused beds on social grounds, simply because the hospitals were full, and returned to deliver in what had been deemed by the midwife to be unsatisfactory domestic surroundings. Furthermore, one district midwife recalled that 'It seemed that the poorer they were ... the more babies they had the less likely they were to agree to a hospital confinement ...' (Allison 1996: 64). A district midwife who worked in Sheffield recalled caring for a woman with several children who gave birth on her kitchen floor looking onto the street. It was not just the socially needy who might refuse hospital confinement; those deemed to be in obstetric need might also do so. By 1959 over 80 per cent of twin births took place in hospital, because they were considered to be risky to mother and babies. Again in Sheffield, one former district midwife who already had four children and suspected (rightly) that she was carrying twins, chose to give birth at home (Mathers and McIntosh 2000). When it actually came down to it, it was impossible to 'force' mothers into hospital births, and women continued to exercise control over their place of birth.

The home/hospital debate expressed a dichotomy that was actually more muddied in real life than on paper, because 'hospitals' were not a monolithic entity. The RCOG may have hankered after huge teaching hospitals, where students could experience every conceivable complication (in 1944 there were calls for 700 maternity beds, covering 14,000 deliveries, simply to train medical students) (*BMJ* 1944). Not only in London, however, but across the country a large proportion of 'institutional' births took place in cottage hospitals, maternity homes and GP units, where there might only be a handful of beds. In 1959, 18 per cent of all beds were in GP units with an average size of 13 beds, although they ranged from 2–50. Their regional spread was varied, with very few in London (an average of 5.4 beds per million population) and a significant amount in areas such as the South-West (160 beds per million population) (Ministry of Health 1959). One of the areas with a high level of GP beds was Oxfordshire, where selected GPs liaised closely with city consultants over the work of GP units. Davis (2011), in her oral history of maternity in Oxfordshire, argued that the specific locality of birth – whether rural or urban, whether the GP carried the respect of the community or not – had as much of an impact on women's experiences of maternity as national debates and policy.

Women's experiences resonated, and had a significant impact on the choices they made. One woman described her home birth in 1948:

> In the end I was very exhausted and the GP told me that he would put me to sleep and that when I awoke 'it would all be over'. It was a forceps delivery as my baby had a large head. When I awoke the GP was stitching me where I had been torn. I was very emotional and cried for no particular reason. Blood was spattered around, even on the wallpaper!
>
> (Devlin 1995: 109)

In many ways this story mirrors that told by the exhausted and frightened GP dealing with forceps and haemorrhage on his own. The sequel for this woman was different, however; she chose to have her second baby in hospital and she described it as a big improvement on the 'ghastly experience' of her first baby. Other women described uncomplicated births in hospital:

> My baby was born in a maternity hospital and it was quite natural, with only gas and air as pain relief. I had a midwife only for the labour and then the doctor came in just before my daughter was born, which seemed to be normal practice.
>
> (Devlin 1995: 109)

This experience is probably representative of what a lot of women experienced at this time: births which were 'managed' but remained low technology and low key. Throughout the period, whatever the other upheavals, midwives continued to deliver around 80 per cent of all babies, and it was this relationship that continued to resonate for the majority of women despite the setting of birth.

Providing analgesia

One of the things about her labour that the woman in the quote above remembered very clearly was the analgesia she had, and it is one of the aspects of labour that women can usually recall with some certainty, even if the memory of exactly what they were given remains hazy. The story of analgesia was linked to the story of the place of birth in the post-war period, and demonstrated some of the same features of professional rivalry, women's agency, and the practicalities of different forms of provision.

Despite an extensive campaign for the expansion of the use of analgesia for labour under the auspices of the National Birthday Trust Fund (NBTF) in the 1930s, very few women had access to pain relief before the Second World War (Williams 1997). The Trust initially called for the provision of anaesthetists by hospitals, but soon switched their attention to the development of a form of analgesia which midwives could use, particularly in domiciliary work. The belief, by Lady Baldwin (founding member and leading light of the NBTF) in particular, that every woman should have access to analgesia met with opposition, perhaps predictably, from GPs who held to themselves the responsibility to provide analgesia where required and not to give further power to the midwife. In practice, however, because GPs did not attend most domiciliary births, most women had no choice about whether to have analgesia or not. Both Williams (1997) and Beinart (1990) argued that for many women, the concept of pain in labour was a largely irrelevant one, because there were so many other more pressing anxieties in life. For some it may have been that the offer of analgesia raised the spectre of the attendance of the doctor, with the fear of instruments and injury that came too. However, it is more likely that in the inter-war period women did not demand pain relief for labour because it was simply not on their radar; pain and labour went together for better or for worse unless you were very rich or very ill.

This was very much the conclusion reached by a survey into maternity conducted by the RCOG in 1944 and reported in 1948, in which it was admitted that the poor status of midwives, the intransigence of doctors, and the belief that pain was a necessary concomitant of labour prevented research into analgesia. In the 1930s different forms of analgesia which could be administered by a midwife were explored and discarded. The method finally approved to be used by midwives was a gaseous mixture of nitrous oxide and air, delivered orally through cumbersome equipment. Its administration and effects were an inexact science due to the uncertainty of the mix; one of the main ways it provided analgesia was through a certain level of hypoxia (lack of oxygen) (Moir 1980). The CMB agreed that midwives should be instructed in its use, but this was taken up only patchily. Some Local Authorities felt it was pointless to train midwives, particularly in rural areas, because the equipment was so difficult to transport; it weighed 22 pounds which made it virtually impossible to carry around (Stocks Report 1949: 26). Furthermore, in the rules laid down for its use, there had to be two midwives present before it could be used; in some areas where one midwife was at a premium, this was a practical impossibility. In consequence, at the outbreak of the Second World War only 29 of the 188 Local Authorities had provided their domiciliary midwives with any training (Williams 1997) and some hospitals, such as the Jessop in Sheffield, refused to have anything to do with the scheme (McIntosh 1997). Throughout the War the situation remained that women either paid for medical aid and the analgesia which came with it, or they booked for a hospital birth, where pain relief was more freely available. Pethidine, a synthetic opioid developed in Germany during the war, was used in 75 per cent of hospital labours by 1948. In contrast midwives working on the district were not able to offer it to their women until 1951.

Commentators have argued that the provision of analgesia for women was another tool of control wielded by the medical profession, since they had decided what could be offered, in what dosage, and when. This left women in a vulnerable position since if they wanted pain relief they had to cede agency. The same issue applied to midwives, particularly those working with home births. The Stocks Report argued that the issue of analgesic provision was one which had to be solved in favour of the district midwife because their inability to offer what women wanted put them in a weak position vis-à-vis both doctors and hospitals (1949: 27). Even when finally permitted to administer pethidine, they were not able to offer it in the higher doses that doctors preferred to use (Roberts 1955) and 'gas and air' was to be offered only in second stage, rather than all the way through labour as was common in hospital settings (Carter 1948). As with other aspects of maternity, the reality was more muddied than this, with practical considerations as significant as philosophical ones. The RCOG survey into maternity in Great Britain (1948) uncovered a wide variation in the provision of gas and air equipment by Local Authorities, regardless of whether they were rural or urban areas. In Croydon over half of all women delivered received analgesia which was transported either by the midwife in her car or by ambulance. In another area surveyed the rate was much lower because the local authority felt the equipment was too heavy to be carried on a bike, but refused to subsidise cars for midwives. Economics, as usual, was therefore an issue.

Economics was also relevant to women themselves; 48 per cent of women who engaged a doctor for delivery received some level of pain relief, compared to 7.6 per cent cared for by midwives (RCOG 1948: 82). Broken down into social class, the Survey suggested that 57.8 per cent of 'professional and salaried' workers received analgesia compared to 18.5 per cent of manual workers (or rather the wives of each group). Women of all classes were beginning to demand analgesia; one was quoted in the Survey as saying, 'Something should be given. I was tired out before I started. People with plenty of money don't have to suffer pain' (RCOG 1948: 80). The evidence suggests that in many cases women were happy to give up a level of control over their labour and birth in order to have relief from pain.

The RCOG felt that never mind doctors gate-keeping access to pain relief, midwives both on the district and in hospital were likely to do the same. Their Survey suggested that women did not receive pain relief unless they were very demanding because it was 'trouble' for the midwife. In the late 1950s a district midwife in Sheffield recalled having to walk to a woman through the snow 'carrying the gas and air machine, the spare cylinder, the antenatal bag, the delivery bag, my bag with my gown and everything else in' (Mathers and McIntosh 2000). Furthermore midwives had to stay with women who were using analgesia; they could not pop in and out, attending to other visits and duties. The use of pain relief therefore impacted on the midwife's workload, whether in the home or the hospital.

Nevertheless, across the period, the use of analgesia by midwives for women increased dramatically. This was partly organisational; after 1946 all pupil midwives had to have a certificate of competency in providing gas and air analgesia before they could be admitted to the Midwives Roll, which meant that more midwives were able to offer pain relief. By 1952, 87 per cent of midwives were trained in its use, and with the increasing provision of cars for midwives, it became a more practical option. In 1949, 43 per cent of women who birthed at home availed themselves of gas and air and by 1952 the proportion had risen to 62 per cent. In some places this took slightly longer: Nottingham City did not start training its midwives to use gas and air until 1948, although by 1952 half of the women delivering at home availed themselves of it (*MoH Reports Nottingham*). Doris, a district midwife in rural Lincolnshire, suggested that women who delivered at home had a better experience of pain relief than those in hospital by the end of the 1950s because their midwife knew them, and had a perception of their needs and limits.

Dealing with pain was not just about the provision of chemical analgesia, however. Early in the period, when the majority of women were calling for the greater availability of pain relief, some were demanding the right to birth in a different way. Much of the impetus for this came from the work of Grantly Dick-Read (1933, 1942) who insisted that if approached in the right frame of mind, labour and birth should be painless. He developed the concept of a fear-tension-pain triad, and argued that if fear could be removed, then labour would be both physiologically easier and psychologically more satisfying. Undoubtedly a man who polarised opinion, he believed that he needed to do no research to back up his claims because his ideas were right (Kitzinger, interview with author). Although he alienated sections of the medical profession with his black and white approach, his ideas were promulgated with some enthusiasm, not just by women, but by doctors, anaesthetists and midwives too (Michael 1952; Roberts 1955; Mathers and McIntosh 2000: 120). This flies in the face of received wisdom that it was groups such as the Natural (later National) Childbirth Trust who championed his ideas in the face of official hostility and derision. In many respects Dick-Read's ideas were not new, but it was the enthusiasm with which he developed them which caught the attention of professionals, and, particularly through the work of Helen Heardman (1951), some members of the public. By 1952 the Ministry of Health was reporting that 'in a small but increasing number of clinics, relaxation techniques are being taught', and midwives recall being involved in similar provision from the mid-1950s.

One of the demands of Grantly Dick-Read and later the National Childbirth Association (afterwards the Natural, and then National Childbirth Trust) was for antenatal classes to prepare women for the experience of labour. This had a two-fold reasoning: it would reduce the fear caused by lack of knowledge about the process and it would enable women to work better with the medical profession. Dick-Read was himself a doctor and his intention was that his methods of relaxation should be used in the hospital rather than the domestic setting. This belief was carried forward by the National Childbirth Association, set up by Patricia Briance in 1956, when it moved to supporting the Lamaze method of preparation for childbirth. Successful use of the method meant that women could labour quietly in a busy hospital, where there might be several women together in one room, and remain receptive to the instructions of their attendants. Women themselves appear to have had little memory regarding antenatal classes of any kind, but some did recall finding their own way to Dick-Read: 'For my first baby I was recommended the book by Grantly Dick-Read, which was full of relaxation advice and breathing techniques. I did practise this and it was a tremendous help I must say. I would have been very nervous and this book gave me confidence' (Devlin 1995: 72). Others took their help from various quarters; Jane, who had her first baby in 1949 read Dick-Read but also described her midwife as 'a fantastic tower of strength to many' (Devlin 1995: 73). Others found his advice useful but tempered by the realities of childbirth: the woman above who found Dick-Read useful commented that 'I had a pethidine injection because I was in terrible pain and it really helped' (Devlin 1995: 110). Women continued to pick and choose the methods they used and the advice they took to get them through labour, and although it has been suggested that the ideas of Dick-Read were ignored until the development of the NCA (Kitzinger 1990), there is no evidence that this was the case.

The original intention of the NCA, as conceived by Briance, was to train sympathetic doctors to teach and use Dick-Read's methods (*The Times* 1957). The linked demand of the Association was that analgesia should only be given if required and not as a matter of course. This was, at the time, a highly contentious statement because in some areas women were only just beginning to have their demands for analgesia realised. To choose nothing was not a position that the majority of women were prepared to take up at this point. However, the NCA always had influence beyond its size, and very soon after its inception Patricia Briance gave evidence to the Cranbrook Committee on the views of women concerning birth in England. The NCA did not represent the broad swathe of women; its members were overwhelmingly middle class and in some cases aristocratic. They occupied the same social space as the doctors they dealt with, and were not cowed by authority in the form of either people or opinions.

That the idea that women were coerced or frightened into hospital births by the scare tactics of doctors was never the whole story. In urban areas, including Nottingham, Birmingham, Sheffield and parts of London, demand for hospital births by women always outstripped the availability of beds. In 1960, there was a debate in London about whether all women should have access to hospital beds; this was not for medical reasons but because women increasingly felt that they were 'entitled' to a hospital bed. The argument was made that women should be allowed to have their babies at home, but not forced to if they preferred hospital, and it was noted that these women tended to be 'highly intelligent and provident women' (*The Times* 12.2.1960). Looking back on the period, campaigner Jean Robinson (interview with the author) argued that it was the 'articulate middle class' who got hospital beds even in times of shortage, because they booked early and believed the rhetoric about safety, and had the confidence to ask for what they wanted. For these women labour and birth was becoming more than a stepping stone to parenthood, but an achievement in itself. For others it is likely that it carried no special mystery and no particular expectations. It is probable, however, that the falling birth rate contributed to the idea that birth had to be special. For women giving birth perhaps only twice in their lifetime, where their mothers had done so five times and their grandmothers ten times, the experience gained a scarcity value. This belief developed over the coming decades and had a significant impact on perceptions.

Conclusion

Kitzinger has suggested that before the NCA childbirth was seen as a private and shameful act, controlled entirely by scaremongering doctors and cold midwives. Certainly these professionals had their own battles to fight, but women continued to have agency throughout the period, over fundamental issues such as the place of birth and the provision of pain relief. The historiography of the period presents a muddled picture, with commentators arguing for, variously, a golden age of home-based midwifery care where women knew and trusted their care givers, to a harsh, fear-driven vision of birth in ignorance. Midwives had a considerable degree of autonomy in their work, but they also often had little semblance of a normal life. Clearly the evidence of women, midwives, obstetricians and GPs demonstrates their different perspectives, but overall the picture was neither as bleak, nor as rosy as historians and commentators have sometimes suggested.

5   1961–80

Introduction

From the 1920s onwards some women and some doctors had been campaigning for birth to take place in the hospital rather than the home. This was argued for a variety of reasons, depending on the standpoint of the protagonist, but was well underway by 1960. The following 20 years saw the triumph of the argument for hospital birth, although it was couched not in terms of the safety of the mother, as had been the case in the inter-war years, or rest from the tribulations of home life. Instead the debate focused on the health of the foetus and on the convenience of organised hospital-based birth to both family and maternity service. This chapter will explore the discovery of the foetus and the explosion in the belief in scientific birth during this period and will discuss the impact that these had on patterns of care. The ubiquity of hospital birth took both women and midwives out of their communities and impacted significantly on their perceptions of maternity. However, professional and consumer groups did not fit easily into pigeon holes and although some midwives disliked and distrusted new ways of working and new technology, others embraced it enthusiastically for a variety of reasons. Similarly, although some women campaigned for a reduction in the use of technology around birth, others campaigned for greater access to new procedures such as epidural anaesthesia. There was a multiplicity of discourses underneath the overriding one which characterised birth as at least potentially pathological, and hospital birth as the desirable norm. However, groups who argued for a different model of care to that which prevailed found themselves increasingly drawn into the mainstream. This chapter will argue that social and class connections between women's groups and doctors in particular gave them unique access to debate and policy around maternity care. It also meant that their arguments were more easily heard and more easily neutralised by the establishment. Despite the work of groups such as the NCT, the regulation and industrialisation of pregnancy and birth continued across the period.

The chapter will consider the rise of scientific birth, and the attitude to it expressed by midwives and women. It will then explore the impact of these debates on the place of birth, as well the work of consumer groups such as the

NCT and AIMS and attempts by policy makers and institutions to 'humanise' birth in a world of machines. Finally it will explore the work of midwives across this period, and the extent to which they and women were able to make common cause in the face of changing patterns of care.

Scientific birth

In a review of the changing emphasis of obstetric care across this period, Schwarz (1990) drew attention to the language used by successive editions of obstetric textbooks. He observed that the choice of words increasingly placed a barrier between doctor and patient, with the language becoming colder and more scientific over time. The period when this shift was most noticeable was that of the 1960s and early 1970s. Midwifery may have still been regarded by many as an art, but obstetrics was positioning itself very much as a science. This section explores the growth and influence of scientific concepts of pregnancy and birth, and the way in which they changed not only the work of obstetricians but the whole debate around maternity. They both fed into, and were influenced by, beliefs and idea around the place of birth and around concepts of safety. Scientific birth went further than that, however, altering how obstetricians characterised their profession, and throwing the contrasts between the services offered by hospital and community services into sharp relief.

The Scottish obstetrician Ian Donald summed up the prevailing mood in the fourth edition of his textbook *Practical Obstetric Problems*:

> The scope of antenatal care is now widening rapidly in two directions; the first, naturally enough, in the field of more sophisticated investigations which are bound to multiply as obstetrics becomes less of an art and more of a science and as it becomes increasingly within our power to estimate the inter-uterine progress of the baby and its development, as well as the welfare of its mother.
>
> (Donald 1972: 1)

This comment brought to the fore the fact that increasingly obstetricians had two potential areas of influence. The interest of obstetricians in the mother, and in particular the mother in labour, dated back hundreds of years. The new part of the equation was the foetus. Historians have argued that the 1960s and 1970s saw the abandonment of interest in the mother in favour of that of the unborn baby, with the pregnant woman becoming little more than a vessel (Shorter 1983). Donald's quote certainly focused on the contribution of antenatal care to foetal, rather than maternal health. He explicitly acknowledged the role of the foetus in obstetric work in the earlier edition of his textbook: 'In place of maternal mortality, perinatal mortality has now become the yardstick by which we review our work. This is at least a sound beginning which acknowledges our custodianship of the baby's future' (Donald 1964: vi).

Obstetrics was no longer to be about heroics performed in the second stage, designed to extract a live baby and healthy mother from a seemingly hopeless situation. Instead it was, as several leading members of the profession described it, to be based on science rather than heroism, and facts rather than gut instinct. Donald himself was no disinterested observer; he was a hands-on obstetrician with a particular interest in the developing field of obstetric ultrasound, which allowed the foetus to be physically 'seen' for the first time and he therefore had a philosophy to promulgate around the centrality of the foetus, as he saw it (Willocks and Barr 2004). The development of ultrasound in the 1960s and early 1970s classically demonstrates several of the features of the 'new' obstetrics. These were the continued significance of the 'heroic' individual researcher, the use of new technologies with little idea as to what benefits they might bring (and no research to back it up), the importance of machines, and rapid spread of their use from specific cases to general surveillance. In common with other obstetric advances, the story of ultrasound has been told very much as a tale of the prowess of individuals, and occasionally a battle with the unenlightened views of colleagues and authority. The picture drawn was one of enthusiastic amateurism and a spirit of enquiry which could overcome all obstacles:

> With his forceful personality, his enthusiasm and his gift for leadership, Donald soon attracted a group of assistants who were willing to work all hours of the day to provide the technical and clinical experience that would get the project up and working.
>
> (Willocks and Barr 2004: 80)

Set piece stories which demonstrated an enterprising spirit and iconoclastic approach were repeated *ad infinitum* in lectures, papers and memoirs (a good example is of Donald and his colleagues taking a selection of removed tumours and a lump of steak for imaging to a local firm who used similar technology to ultrasound for detecting flaws in metal (Willocks and Barr 2004: 70)). Their research, which suggested that areas such as pregnancy diagnosis and gestational age, as well as foetal size and position could be determined by ultrasound, was presented to the Royal Society in 1962. As a colleague of Donald's remarked, many of the audience 'had never heard of diagnosis by ultrasound and many remained incredulous' (Willocks and Barr 2004: 85). Such incredulity allowed individual obstetricians to present themselves as pioneering explorers. Obstetricians did not speak with one voice; they could be fiercely critical of each other and of different ideas, and very protective of their own beliefs. An example of this attitude can be seen in Donald's views about another developing area of practice: induction of labour. He argued very forcefully that '... no method of induction is certain and safe ... What is more surprising is that, on the whole, the results of induction are as good as they are. It remains, nevertheless, one of the most abused procedures in all obstetrics' (Donald 1964: 348).

Other colleagues may well have made similar comments about the development of ultrasound. Clearly the emergence of new ideas and technologies flourished across the period for a number of reasons. RCOG had an increasing professional confidence born of such reports as the *Perinatal Mortality Survey* (Butler and Bonham 1963), which demonstrated that their views and ideas were taken very seriously by policy makers. The way that the NHS was set up left all consultants, whatever their speciality, with a significant power base and sphere of influence, not least in relation to their junior staff, patients and policy makers. Obstetricians were no exception, and having traditionally always been perceived as rather a lowly group in the hierarchy of medicine, they were now poised to flex their professional muscles. There was also an element of professional need in their desire to develop new techniques and technologies. With the exception of forceps, progress in obstetrics had been made through the application of the work of others (antibiotics, blood transfusion) rather than as a result of the efforts of obstetricians themselves. Childbirth remained uniquely hard to control, with there still being little understanding of how and why labour even started, for example. Apart from anything else, this meant that obstetricians, unlike their colleagues in other specialities, never got to escape the threat of night and weekend duty, even if in practice they left much of the work to their juniors. New technologies such as ultrasound, which initially proved most successful in obstetrics after a failure to impress in other specialities, gave obstetricians the chance to make their own claims for greatness and to push back their sphere of influence deep into pregnancy. In many ways such developments allowed them to rewrite their job descriptions, becoming not just operators of instruments to end a difficult labour, but laying the claim to be an indispensable professional adjunct to the whole of pregnancy.

Initially there seem to have been few claims made for the benefits of ultrasound, other than for the thrill of seeing the previously invisible. It was suggested that foetal growth could be tracked, or gross foetal abnormalities detected, but no mention was made of how these achievements might alter the management of pregnancy. The effort put into developing better ultrasound pictures or more manoeuvrable equipment was not reflected in its initial use, although it demonstrated the unacknowledged importance of tie-ups between technology companies and obstetricians in this and other areas. This linkage would naturally lead to the desire to have machines bought by hospitals, since their development represented an outlay in time and effort by both the companies themselves and their medical bedfellows. Beyond the practicalities, however, the development of the ability to 'see' through ultrasound, or manipulate through induction was a powerful, if unacknowledged, incentive. It was in this period that the French philosopher Foucault (2003) developed his ideas of medical hegemony specifically through what he described as the 'clinical gaze'. It was in this particular way of seeing and codifying the vagaries of the human body that the doctor put himself above others. The development of ultrasound meant that obstetricians would not have to rely on what women were telling them; doctors could now tell women, everything from the date they conceived, the position of their baby and the date it would (or should) be born. This would have a powerful impact on relations between doctors and women.

The concept of foetal health, or more accurately, foetal surveillance, was not left entirely in the hands of doctors. It also attracted the attention of midwives, particularly those working in the hospital setting and able to watch it develop at first hand. Just as medical textbooks reflected changing mores, so did midwifery textbooks, with *Mayes' Midwifery* including a chapter on foetal health in 1972, when in the previous edition of 1967 there had been nothing (Bailey 1972). Margaret Myles' textbook, which saw three editions in the 1960s alone, charted the developments in the debate around the emerging technologies: 'Midwives must comprehend and be equipped to assist with new diagnostic techniques and clinical procedures: the need for more scientific observation of the foetal condition during labour demands familiarity with the mechanical devices now employed ...' (Myles 1968: v).

In the fourth edition of 1961, the section on induction of labour contained a variety of caveats: 'the routine varies in different hospitals'; 'intramuscular injections are occasionally given'; 'not all are agreed on this'. In the sixth edition, which appeared in 1968, these qualifications were gone to be replaced by instructions which brooked no debate. The author did admit, however, that 'Recent advances in the field of obstetrics have been so numerous and opinions regarding them so diverse that presenting to midwives a balanced account of current thought and methods of treatment has been no easy task' (Myles 1968: v).

By 1975 even this caveat was gone and the suggested indications for induction of labour had mushroomed to include all primigravidae over 30 years of age who were at term. Myles now argued that 'It is logical and humane that the expectant mother should share the benefits of induced labour now that it has proved a safe and effective procedure for mother and fetus.' This logic was extended to cover not only the issue of expected improved physical safety, but also the psychological benefits:

> The unpredictability of the expected date of delivery is eliminated so the woman can plan the care of her children: the husband can arrange to be on holiday: worry over reaching the hospital on time is precluded.
>
> The woman has a much shorter labour, 8 to 12 hours or less: prolonged labour and disordered uterine action are not permitted to occur: no harm to mother or fetus ensues. Modern intensive care now considered essential during labour can be provided more effectively during the day when senior doctors are readily available. The use of automated infusion units, the need for skilful administration of pain relieving drugs: the use of monitors which enhance maternal and fetal safety demand supervision by thoroughly experienced senior midwives. This aspect of obstetric care is highly specialised and many labour ward sisters are extremely competent in using the modern equipment that extends their powers of observation as well as enabling women to have short, comfortable and safe labours.
>
> (Myles 1975: 549)

This quote demonstrates several features of changing maternity practice. The first is that midwives did not necessarily see themselves as losing midwifery skills in the service of high-technology birth, but rather as gaining a whole series of new ones. Beyond this, however, was the belief that birth could and should be controlled, not just for reasons of safety, but for equally compelling social reasons. Control was not just to be vested in the 'senior doctor' more readily available in the day time, but also to women and their partners who would no longer be at the whim of the raw biological process of birth. This issue of control was exhibited in its most pure form through 'active management of labour', a concept initially developed at the Rotunda Hospital in Dublin under its Master Kieran O'Driscoll, but quickly exported to Britain (O'Driscoll et al. 1973; O'Driscoll and Meagher 1980). By 1979 Donald had altered the title of his chapter on 'prolonged labour' which appeared in 1972 to 'management of labour'. As Myles' quote demonstrated, watchful waiting was now seen as tantamount to neglect and whereas in previous editions of *Practical Obstetric Problems*, Donald had been content to suggest that labours lasting over 36 hours were 'to some extent abnormal' (1972: 504), by 1979, he stated firmly that 'Dawn should not rise twice upon the same labour' (1979: 563). The chapter itself was completely rewritten to take account of this development in philosophy and the belief that labour should last no longer than six to twelve hours. In order to accomplish this, oxytocic drugs and concomitant intensive monitoring were employed from an early stage in the belief that 'Nature left to her own devices often fails to achieve the pattern and duration of labour which we now accept as normal' (1979: 575). This 'normality' included keeping the patient nil by mouth, and in O'Driscoll's (1973) model, with the constant attendance of a midwife who meticulously recorded every development on the newly developed pictorial partogram (Philpott 1972; Studd 1973). Friedman curves (1967) for indentifying normal, and abnormal, progress in labour, together with partograms which gave a graphical representation of all physical aspects of a labour, allowed obstetricians and midwives a sense of control. They also contributed to the belief that there were patterns in a normal labour which could be identified, and that any deviations from these could and should be corrected.

The development of writing in the main midwifery textbooks suggested that midwives saw themselves as having a professional stake in any obstetric developments; there is a sense that midwives should not get left behind in the rush to technology. Textbooks only gave a partial picture of what was happening in reality, but they are likely to have exerted a powerful influence at a time when midwifery teachers taught from one of the main textbooks, and students were expected to learn from it (Diane interview; Maureen interview). For many midwives the new machinery and new ideas were as exciting as they were for doctors. More recently midwives have decried technology and the impact that it has had on their role as perceived guardians of normality (Robinson 1990; Walsh 2007). However, midwives were not in the vanguard of the fight against technology, and on an individual as well as institutional level many embraced it:

> Induction of labour for everyone and all these wonderful monitors ... utterly bizarre but I think it was regarded as progress, but retrospectively, you can't think that there was anything very normal about any of it, but it was the progressive way to manage labour ... it was actually quite early on in the technology and some of it was quite pioneering, I think.
>
> (Jane interview)

Brenda commented on the effect she saw technology having on relations between hospital and district midwives:

> And then we'd got the Sonicaids [handheld ultrasound monitors for hearing the foetal heartbeat] which were obviously brilliant. But I think that's where the hospital midwives differed from the community mid-wives. They were highly technically qualified. We had the experience but obviously we didn't have the technology that they'd been taught. And I think that probably all midwives should have gone in to be taught the technology of it all, so that you could interchange at any time, you could have a community midwife able to go in.
>
> (Brenda interview)

There was a growing sense over the period, articulated by Brenda, that the two midwifery roles were diverging faster than ever. Midwives who had worked on the district spoke of how de-skilled they felt if they returned to work in a hospital and were faced with new machines and unfamiliar procedures:

> ... because everybody was on a monitor, everybody, and then the monitor would stop. 'Oh God, there's something wrong again,' and you'd go or you'd ring the bell. 'Oh don't worry about that, it does that sometimes.' ... and I thought how do you know when it's happening for real?
>
> (Brenda interview)

For those midwives who worked in the hospital setting, however, the picture looked very different. One midwife recalled that after working at University College Hospital in London, which was developing some of the new technology in use, she moved to a quieter suburban hospital. She found the lack of invest-ment in technology strange, and argued that the hospital felt backward and old-fashioned in comparison to what she was used to (Diane interview). Another midwife who worked in Manchester in the mid-1960s described how the hospital where she worked was one of the first to have an electronic foetal heart monitor:

> ... and I understood it to be only the second one in the country, a labour monitor. The Simpson Memorial [hospital] had one in Edinburgh and we got one. The transducers were great, we used to strap them on, one for

the contractions and one for the foetal heart and they were monstrous things. Of course, it was quite exciting because we'd never seen a foetal heart monitor before ... I thought everybody should have the benefit of this technology.

(Stella interview)

As she explained, the sense of excitement extended beyond the midwives themselves:

I know when I was head of midwifery somebody approached me to raise some money, it was a women's organisation, could even have been the Soroptomists I think, and we really needed a foetal pulse detector. They bought it, they came and presented it to me and I demonstrated it ... and they were just in raptures about this. They weren't patients, they were mainly older women, but it was something they'd never seen.

(Stella interview)

If the technology to allow scientific births was new and exciting, it was also a very scarce resource. Most women birthing in hospitals did not have access to foetal heart monitors, for example, during this period. The equipment was cumbersome and expensive, and initially at least, was reserved for a tiny minority of women. Stella described a particular anaesthetist in the teaching hospital where she worked who wanted to 'try' a new anaesthetic technique called an epidural. On his day on labour suite he would do one epidural. She did not describe how the guinea pig was selected or to what extent women had choices over such interventions.

Commenting on rising induction rates across the period, Stella said:

Well we had a number we could manage ... I don't know what the number was but say it was seven a day, that was all we could give adequate care to because of course we'd got the other spontaneous labours coming in. There's a place for induction isn't there?

(Stella interview)

The place of birth

The development and increasing use of technology did not happen in a vacuum. Advances were sometimes related more to the interests of individuals than the wider demands of the profession or of the public. Nevertheless debates around the increasing use of technology tended to be linked to wider discussions around safety and risk which gathered pace throughout this period. These in turn fostered continued argument about the best setting for birth to take place.

Arguably the biggest influence on rhetoric and policy in the 1960s and 1970s was the *Perinatal Mortality Survey*, a joint venture between the NBTF and RCOG (Butler and Bonham 1963). Although it reported after the Cranbrook Report, which had pledged the government to continuing, if nebulous, support for homebirth, the survey on which the *Perinatal Mortality Survey* was based was actually carried out in 1958. Once published, in 1963, the Report changed both the landscape of maternity services and the terms of the debate. Some writers have argued that the *Perinatal Mortality Survey* signalled the decisive shift of the focus of official and medical interest from mother to child (Shorter 1983). As the work of obstetricians such as Donald demonstrated, this move was largely recognised at the time. However, the shift in emphasis had a significant impact on the wider philosophy and practicalities of maternity care.

The statistician Marjorie Tew, working in the 1980s, effectively demolished one of the central planks of the Report which stated that hospitals were not only the safest places for women to give birth but also the safest places for babies to be born (Campbell and Macfarlane 1990; Tew 1995). Her broad conclusions were generally accepted by health professionals and policy makers, and informed some of the changes in the debate which would occur in the 1990s. As far as the *Perinatal Mortality Survey* was concerned, the evidence was demonstrated by Tew not to have supported some of the wide ranging conclusions reached by the Report. However, despite the validity, or otherwise, of its claims, the Report was taken up enthusiastically by obstetricians seeking to further develop a hospital-based maternity service, and as we have already seen through the Cranbrook Report, their beliefs and recommendations carried weight with policy makers. It was this aspect which was to give the Report its lasting impact because it appeared to give powerful support to the argument that hospital birth, under the management of an obstetrician, was the safest environment in which to have a baby; a concept not challenged until the 1980s by which time virtually all babies were born in hospital. Beyond the headlines, however, the Report demonstrated that whatever front they might present in newspapers or to government bodies, obstetricians were divided about best practice. Types of care and intervention varied across hospitals and between regions. Hospital deliveries were highest in London and the South-East with 58.6 per cent of births taking place in institutions. In the neighbouring Southern region the rate was at its lowest with 27.1 per cent of births in hospital. London had a high concentration of teaching hospitals, both for doctors and midwives, and a long-standing commitment to the development and use of technology. For women who delivered in hospital, their practical experience was different to that of those who stayed at home. They were more likely to have pain relief, but they were also more likely to have other interventions.

One area highlighted by the *Perinatal Mortality Survey* which illustrated the increasingly divergent birthing practices seen at home and in hospital, and the changing work of midwives, was around the use of episiotomy (the cutting of the perineum as the baby's presenting part birthed). Some 41.2 per cent of women having their first baby in hospital had an episiotomy compared with 11.3 per cent in domiciliary practice; and this was occurring before the belief in the liberal use of episiotomy became fashionable in Britain, although it had been a long-standing feature of practice in the USA (Graham 1997). The relatively low rate of episiotomies in domestic practice was linked to the fact that midwives were allowed to perform neither them nor any perineal repair. For district midwives, therefore, an intact perineum was to be striven for since anything else would necessitate the call out of the GP. Margaret, who worked as a district midwife during this period, recalled the importance to midwives of a careful delivery technique to try and ensure an intact perineum, 'You would help by feeling underneath to try and help that head to come up, because the rectum just opens, doesn't it, and you can help the head to come up and very slowly' (Margaret interview).

It was not until 1967 that the CMB authorised the use of episiotomies by midwives in emergency situations. Although the use of episiotomies took hold in hospital practice in the 1970s, and midwives were increasingly expected to perform one as the head crowned, they were still required to defer to doctors on the question of repair. Midwives were not permitted to undertake perineal suturing for either tears or episiotomies until 1983 (Graham 1997).

The use of episiotomies by midwives could be regarded as a bellwether in the move from home to hospital and the loss of autonomous midwifery practice. Mary Renfrew, a midwife and midwifery researcher who trained in the late 1970s, recalled that by this point all first-time mothers had an episiotomy. Looking back she linked this explicitly to the primacy of obstetricians over hospital care, and the lack of control which midwives had over the way that they worked (Graham 1997: 76). At the time, however, she agreed that the change 'swept over the midwifery profession very fast' and Diane, another midwife who trained earlier in the 1970s, recalled that the idea of an episiotomy protecting both the baby's head and preventing more serious perineal injuries 'seemed to make sense' (interview). By 1978 53.4 per cent of all births included an episiotomy; the high point for the procedure (Kitzinger and Simkin 1986; Graham 1997; Mugford and Macfarlane 2000).

In 1970 the Peel Report was published by the government. The Standing Maternity and Midwifery Advisory Committee had been convened in order to address the outcomes, some unintended, which the *Perinatal Mortality Survey* had led to, principally around the increasing vexed question of the provision of a domiciliary service and the perceived need for institutional maternity beds. The expansion in hospital-based maternity services which it had recommended meant that, as the overall birth rate fell, home births were increasingly seen as a costly extravagance. The Report looked at the future provision of a domiciliary service, and the provision of hospital beds, both issues predicated on the belief that hospital was the best place for birth to occur. Its most famous comment, repeated down the years by supporters and opponents of hospital birth, was that:

We consider that the resources of modern medicine should be available to all mothers and babies, and we think that sufficient facilities should be

> provided to allow for 100% hospital delivery. The greater safety of hospital confinement for mother and child justifies this objective.
>
> (Peel Report 1970: 60)

This was the pure essence of the arguments of RCOG and the published results of the *Perinatal Mortality Survey*. Several commentators have argued that the power of the residual fear of maternal mortality still coloured the beliefs and actions of many doctors at this time, and there was almost a sense of resentment by obstetricians that the wider 'folk memory' of maternal death had disappeared from society by the 1970s (Christie and Tansey 2001). One obstetrician who worked through the period commented that 'The impression that I have got from watching my teachers, both obstetricians and midwives, is that these cases, watching somebody die, have a huge impact on the carer and therefore, you know, it changes practice' (Christie and Tansey 2001: 12). The sense was that in individual units it was not the drift of statistics that changed practice, but the impact that one maternal death could have (Christie and Tansey 2001: 21).

However, although the idea of 'home' and 'hospital' conjures up two completely opposing paradigms of belief and care, with hospital care seen as highly technological and medical, and home birth as organic and social in model, the picture was actually more muddled than that throughout the 1960s. As the Peel Report noted, the headline rise in hospital birth rates from 64 to 87 per cent was actually driven by not just the continued survival, but the vigorous expansion of GP maternity beds. In many areas these were seen as the most cost-effective solution to the problems of maternity care provision. Obstetricians might be demanding more hospital beds, and women might be voting with their feet and booking hospital births, but what they were actually getting was more beds in nursing homes or cottage hospitals under the auspices of the much-maligned generalist GP-obstetrician. The fact that 'hospitals' were not a monolithic entity is often forgotten in the debate about the swing from home to hospital care in the 1960s. Between 1955 and 1968, beds in GP units rose by 82.8 per cent, in comparison to beds in consultant units (both district hospitals and teaching hospitals) which grew by only 4.3 per cent. Cities such as Nottingham, as well as rural areas such as Suffolk, struggled for logistical and financial reasons to raise the numbers of consultant beds, and continued to rely on GP beds and domiciliary midwifery for the maintenance of their maternity service. Several participants to the *Wellcome Witness Seminar* into maternal care (Christie and Tansey 2001) drew attention to the success and popularity of these units. As with every aspect of maternity there was, however, an undercurrent, with some midwives feeling that GP units eroded their autonomy, which eventually opened the door to the blanket hospitalisation of birth for low-risk women (Christie and Tansey 2001: 27–29).

Overall, however, the picture was clear. By 1968 there were more than double the numbers of midwives working in hospital as opposed to domestic practice. Although the Peel Report set the tone for the following decade, in many ways it was just codifying what was already occurring, to varying degrees, across the country. Home birth was increasingly seen as a possibly selfish indulgence, and hospital birth had cemented its place as the 'normal' place of delivery for all women:

> To suggest that we should go back to the days of 'home confinement' is like asking a modern surgeon to remove an appendix on the kitchen table. Undoubtedly most of his patients would survive the experience but there would be a few who because of a lack of specialised facilities would suffer.
>
> (*The Times* 06.09.1974)

Complicated assessments of obstetric and social risk became less relevant as the concept of birth as only normal in retrospect became increasingly accepted. This change can be charted not just through statistics, but through changes in textbooks, in the working lives of midwives and in the reproductive experiences of women. Although in the fourth edition of *Myles Midwifery*, published in 1961, 'home confinement' was relegated to a chapter at the end of the book, it did begin by saying that:

> There is little doubt that a woman's own home is the ideal place for her confinement if there are no obstetrical, medical or domestic reasons to the contrary. A home confinement places childbirth in its true perspective as a normal event in a woman's life.
>
> (Myles 1961: 650)

Despite the caveats about risk, home confinement was seen as an integral part of life. By 1975 and the eighth edition of her work, Myles no longer carried the comment that home confinement was normal or desirable and the preface to the edition had admitted that the chapter on home confinement had been severely curtailed as it was virtually obsolete. The concept of risk loomed large with contra-indications including such factors as 'destitution, insanitary conditions, multiple pregnancy and multiparity' which had been warned against 15 years previously. Risk factors now included all primigravidae over 30 years of age, and all multiparous women over 35. Bailey explained succinctly in *Mayes' Midwifery* published in 1976 that 'Home delivery may thus be considered only for a healthy woman under 35, expecting her second or third child, if her previous obstetric history is normal, her present pregnancy uncomplicated and her home suitable' (Bailey 1976: 406).

Much of the change was undoubtedly to do with the belief in the greater safety of hospital birth, and of the efficacy of technology which could only be offered in an institutional setting. It is, therefore, easy to see the Peel Report and the torrent of obstetric interventions of the 1970s as an expression of patriarchal, male, power in its purest form. Women, both as mothers and midwives, were powerless in the face of a self-confident and determined obstetrician. As Caroline Flint, a midwife during this period, observed:

Obstetricians are very self-confident and they expect people to do what they say. And so you have midwives going, you know, hearing what … these very important powerful men were saying … and she [the midwife] would no more challenge this great man than fly to the moon.

(Graham 1997: 78)

Flint was describing specifically the practice of episiotomy but she could have been talking about induction, electronic foetal monitoring and the limitation on lengths of labour, or any of the other interventions increasingly seen as routine elements of care.

In 1979, across the General Election which removed Labour and brought in the Conservatives under Margaret Thatcher, a new committee sat, tasked with exploring the apparently shocking high rate of perinatal and neonatal mortality in England. The Short Report which was published in 1980 commented explicitly on its background as one where 'mounting public concern that babies were unnecessarily dying or suffering permanent damage during the latter part of pregnancy and the earliest part of infancy' (1980: 1). This very emotive language set the tone for the Report which looked not only at mortality figures but at the whole structure of maternity services in England. As far as home births and isolated GP units (those not physically close to consultant services) were concerned the picture it painted was stark. Although the evidence suggested that mothers liked GP units, and may have chosen to birth at home if a distant consultant unit was the only option, the Report argued that both they and home births should be further phased out. This was despite evidence presented that suggested that GP units actually had the lowest mortality rates. The involvement by GPs in intra-partum care had been dealt its final blow, and not just by RCOG but also by the RCM and CMB who agreed that GP units were dangerous (Curzen and Mountrose 1976). However, as with previous reports, the Short Report was in many ways merely codifying what was already occurring. The number of isolated GP units in England had dropped from 226 in 1973 to 151 in 1978, after having risen throughout the 1960s, and the proportion of births that took place in them stood at only 5.7 per cent of total births (Short Report 1980: 26). This partly reflected the accumulation of GPs' lack of confidence in their obstetric skills; despite a rearguard action by GPs such as Luke Zander, most GPs had absorbed the idea that they had neither the time nor expertise to devote to maternity work. Although they still saw women antenatally, the involvement of the vast majority of GPs in intra-partum work was now negligible.

When talking of intra-partum care the Short Report continued to use the powerful language which it had employed in the introduction, suggesting that any perinatal death was a 'failure of obstetric care' and that the labour suite environment should be regarded as analogous with that of an intensive care unit. Women's choice would necessarily have to be sacrificed on the altar of safety, which the Report concluded meant full-time obstetric consultant, anaesthetic and paediatric cover and the full panoply of 'essential' equipment such as electronic foetal heart monitors, ultrasound and blood gas monitoring facilities (1980: 90). Amongst all the high-technology equipment and medical leadership, however, the Report did note the impact that changing patterns of care were having on midwifery. It argued that midwifery should still be regarded as a separate profession, and that the redevelopment of direct entry training should be explored. It stopped short of suggesting that midwives were autonomous professionals, foregrounding instead the importance of 'team work' but it did call for the development of midwifery research, and supported the creation of research career pathways for midwives. Despite the extreme negativity with which the Short Report has always been viewed by midwives (and indeed by a new generation of policy makers), it did make some important points about the development of a research-based service. Although many of its conclusions were predicated on out-dated or misinterpreted data, the Report recognised the need for a better standard of research across the whole service, calling for enquiry into the efficacy of specific areas such as antenatal care, and asking for the Medical Research Council and universities to take an active part in developing and supporting research. This was a new departure, and one which, despite the headlines garnered about the near outlawing of GP and home births, would in future impact significantly on direction and debate in maternity.

Throughout the period there was a multiplicity of voices running through debates on the maternity services. Women continued to demand hospital births, and it was their voices, rather than those of obstetricians, which led initially to the increase in numbers of beds and in changing patterns of care. Mavis, a midwife in Sheffield, described the continued attraction of the hospital environment:

> On the whole I think they [the women] liked it because you got looked after, you got fed and the Jessops [hospital for women] actually had single rooms, it was quite a breakthrough as a building. So you got a private room and you got waited on for, well, a week if you had a normal delivery and ten days if you had a section, and this was the only rest for the next twenty years for many of them.
>
> (Mavis interview)

What did women want?

By 1960 the NCT was no longer the only group in existence which claimed to represent child-bearing women. The Association for Improvements in the Maternity Services (AIMS) was set up by Sally Willington in response to a specific experience and with a specific and challenging remit:

> In hospital, as a matter of course presumably, mothers put up with loneliness, lack of sympathy, lack of privacy, lack of consideration, poor food, unlikely visiting hours, callousness, regimentation, lack of instruction, lack of

rest, deprivation of the new baby, stupidly rigid routines, rudeness, a complete disregard of mental care or of the personality of the mother. Our maternity hospitals are often unhappy places with memories of unhappy experiences. They are overcrowded, understaffed and inhuman. Improvements will involve some rebuilding (more money) and an entirely new attitude to be taught to trainee midwives. If anyone else agrees with me and thinks that something should be done, I hope they will write to me and join the SPCPW (The Society for the Prevention of Cruelty to Pregnant Women).

(The Guardian 01.04.1960)

Both Willington and Patricia Briance, who set up the NCT, had personal experience of hospital maternity care, both came from comfortable intellectual middle-class backgrounds, and were comfortable using the language of 'rights'. Briance later argued that 'You cannot possibly imagine what it was like back then in the fifties, we knew nothing about having a baby and there was no one to tell us; no books or magazines that told you what to expect' (*The Independent* 26.04.1996). Making no mention of midwives or of doctors, she offered a view that was not only stark but that reflected a particular agenda. A woman would expect to get information herself, not rely on professionals; both AIMS and the NCT developed the concept of women not as *patients* but as *consumers* of the maternity services. From the beginning, AIMS in particular was adept at harnessing the power of argument whether through letters to MPs, evidence to local committees, or talks to women's groups. It boasted as members school teachers and welfare workers as well as consultants, surgeons and psychologists, and was granted an audience at the House of Commons just a year after coming into being (*The Times* 06.02.1961). Similarly, the NCT was good at making and using its contacts. In 1963 an interview with Betty Parsons, a teacher with the NCT commented on the 'cordial relationship she has built up within the medical profession' and a book she wrote on antenatal exercises had a 'very complimentary' foreword by John Peel, the President of RCOG who was later to Chair the committee calling for hospital beds to be available to all women (*The Times* 01.04.1963). As Sheila Kitzinger – another childbirth campaigner and wife of an Oxford don – remarked in interview, it was the relationships with doctors that meant things got done and she commented very favourably on relations between herself and the obstetricians at the John Radcliffe Hospital in Oxford. Jean Robinson, who campaigned against what she and others regarded as unnecessary inductions of labour in the 1970s through AIMS, also spoke of her contacts; consultants in both London and Oxford (interview). Clearly, socially these women were on the same level as the doctors and politicians they dealt with and contacts could be informal and non-threatening.

The same often applied to the women who joined the NCT and AIMS, or who used their services. One of the primary functions of the NCT was to run antenatal classes in relaxation and childbirth preparation for women and their partners. As Betty Parsons commented, many of the lessons she gave were private one-to-one lessons; even the group sessions cost money. Choosing to take lessons in natural or active birth was a huge commitment for women not just in terms of money, but time as well. One commentator explained in 1964 that a course of classes usually consisted of eight two-hour sessions, plus daily practice, in order to be properly 'trained' (*The Times* 06.04.1964). This clearly was out of the reach of many women. The same commentator explained, rather scathingly, that although some classes were beginning to be offered on the NHS, a couple of sessions were not going to replicate the intensity needed to achieve success. The issue of power and control is clear during the early years of both AIMS and the NCT. Women were only allowed to attend NCT classes if they had the permission of their doctor; classes were designed to allow women to work with their care givers, not to challenge them, and were predicated on birth taking place in an institutional setting.

In an interview Sheila Kitzinger used the language of control to describe the types of woman attending NCT classes: 'Mostly educated women. Women who were concerned about taking control of their lives and often it wasn't just childbirth but other areas too that they were concerned with.' Kitzinger also described the process of engagement with policy because she argued that real progress came through the media and through government. She described learning to '... manage the media is a bit strong but learning to communicate with the media and express yourself with the media is a specific skill ...' She also talked about putting pressure on Parliament, and getting questions asked by MPs about maternity policy. These were all particular class and social skills, and relied on articulate middle-class women with social skills and contacts to promulgate them. Although campaigners like Kitzinger and Jean Robinson argued that the work they did made a difference to all women, they were putting forward a particular agenda based around the needs and expectations of a particular group of women.

The NCT and AIMS both developed a more radical agenda in the 1970s and 1980s when they increasingly argued against the use of technology, but this was not evident in the early years of either organisation (Kitzinger 1990). Although safety was always central to the rhetoric of the maternity services, and was particularly used to promote hospital birth and the use of technology, gradually certain groups of women began to use different criteria to inform their experience of pregnancy and birth. This was partly based on personal experiences of technologically mediated birth, but the language of feminism seems also to have been significant to many women in terms of the rights and control that they demanded over their own bodies. Equally important was the drive by some women for birth to be seen as a psychological event as much as a physical one.

The argument was not, however, all in one direction. Throughout the 1960s in particular, demand for hospital beds continued to outstrip supply as it had done for the previous three decades. This caused not only philosophical debate but practical strains on the service, particularly with the reduction in hospital stays to 48 hours or less (*The Times* 02.08.1962, 31.10.1962). General practitioners, some of whom were openly accusing obstetricians of empire building over their calls for the effective outlawing of home birth, warned that the drive towards hospitalisation might cause more problems than it solved by pushing the workload and facilities beyond capacities (*The Times* 09.11.1962). Women themselves continued to have agency, calling for the right not only to birth in hospital, but equally to have access to emerging technologies; particularly those relating to pain relief (*The Observer* 19.02.1961; *The Guardian* 12.04.1973).

The development of the use of induction of labour and the active management of birth became one of the flashpoints in the increasing radicalisation of women over maternity issues (Christie and Tansey 2001: 47). The proportion of births induced rose from 15 per cent in 1965 to 41 per cent by 1974 (Cartwright 1979: 1). Women had newspaper reports to draw on which described in detail the use of oxytocics, analgesics and forceps combined to complete labour and delivery within eight hours. This was presented very much as a positive step: 'The consequence of these aids is a shortening of all stages of labour, less pain for the mother and full recovery "within twelve hours" ... The use of procedures that speed delivery can be justified not only to spare the mother exhaustion but to avoid physical stress to the foetus' (*The Times* 25.11.1971, see also: 20.7.1973; Tacchi 1971). Some of the concerns about the wholesale use of oxytocics, such as that they resulted in higher frequency of neonatal jaundice for example, gradually began to creep into medical literature in the early 1970s (Ghosh and Hudson 1972; Campbell et al. 1975). They were not, however, widely reflected in the lay Press. Women, however, increasingly had their own experiences and those of others on which to draw as induction of labour became more and more common across the country. In 1975 Jean Robinson, the Chair of the Patients' Association and a member of AIMS, opened the floodgates with the publication of a report about induction in *The Lancet*. She argued that none of the new obstetric measures took into account the wishes of women or their feelings about having their labour and birth rendered increasingly 'unnatural'. Robinson used detailed correspondence from women on the subject of induction to make her argument, suggesting that although some were appreciative of the service others were left feeling shocked, angry and unprepared for motherhood. Her analysis appeared in national newspapers as well as medical journals, giving it wide lay coverage (*The Times* 12.08.1974). The argument she came up with was a potentially hugely radical one: that women did not see the outcome of pregnancy in purely physical terms:

> Whereas doctors, understandably and properly, judge quality of treatment by peri-natal and maternal mortality rates they may not fully have understood that mothers also judge maternity care in terms of the quality of relationship fostered between them and their babies, and they may even be willing to take greater physical risks to ensure this.
>
> (*The Times* 12.08.1974)

She also drew attention to the impact of induction on the mental health of women, and described some of the letters she received as reminding her of accounts of First World War shell shock cases (Christie and Tansey 2001: 47). Robinson's work provoked considerable interest among obstetricians, some of it couched in very strident tones, with a denigration of her survey by one obstetric professor as merely 'anecdotal' and therefore not worthy of serious regard (*The Times* 22.08.1974). The paternalistic attitude of some of the comments on Robinson's work muddied the waters of the debate by conflating issues of induction with those of home birth and the diminution of the district midwifery service (*The Times* 26.08.1974, 29.08.1974, 04.09.1974, 06.09.1974). The debate led to questions being asked in the House of Commons, particularly around the question of the extent to which hospitals were using induction to manage their workloads over Christmas-time (*The Guardian* 10.12.1974, 13.12.1974; *The Times* 20.12.1974). Obstetricians did not necessarily see any of these issues as inherently problematic; Theobald, who worked in Bradford, was described as offering induction to women not just as a way of giving his working life some order, but as a way of giving women control. He offered multi-parous women induction over the weekend while their husbands looked after the children, and promised that they would be home on Monday morning (Christie and Tansey 2001: 42). Macfarlane (1979), who alongside Tew was one of the first researchers to critique long-accepted maternity statistics around risk and safety, suggested that births were less likely to occur at weekends and bank holidays in the 1970s.

Policy makers made the not altogether unfair point that debates around the use and abuse of induction of labour were being driven by a small section of the child-bearing population. Mersey Regional Health Authority's specialist in community medicine commented that the majority of patients were happy with the situation as it stood and that 'It is the upper middle class woman who wants to do her own thing; they are the ones who are protesting about the interference with natural childbirth. It is different when one is dealing with the ordinary working class mother who is delighted to get it over with' (*The Guardian* 10.12.1974). Evidence from Cartwright, a sociologist who conducted research into women's experiences of induction, found that women from lower social classes were actually less likely to be admitted to hospital in pregnancy or to be offered induction than their middle-class counterparts, despite the fact that they may have had obstetric indications which might warrant intervention such as poorer nutritional status (1979: 30). Similar experiences were reported by women from ethnic minorities (Phoenix 1990). This suggests that middle-class women had a qualitatively different experience of pregnancy and birth to lower-class women, and that the arguments that campaigners advanced were only applicable to a particular section of society. There was clearly, however, an element of paternalism evident in the maternity services, directed particularly at middle-class women, and against which some of them kicked. One of the doctors researching the issue of toxaemia, a dangerous and little understood condition which still carried a potentially fatal risk, commented in terms reminiscent of his Victorian forebears that it was women's refusal to take heed of their biology that caused them problems:

> Toxaemic mothers don't seem to exist as much among the very rich and the very poor. The poor mum stays at home, the rich mother has help. It's the middle class wife who is rushing off to university, eating buns for lunch and trying to do without help in the house that gets into trouble with toxaemia.
>
> *(The Times* 26.08.1970)

Alongside the growing concept of consumerism which argued that women were entitled to have demands and expectations from the service they received, was the vexed thread of feminism. Many second-wave feminists, including writers such as Germaine Greer, argued that motherhood itself should have no place in the life of a thinking woman, and that biology was certainly not destiny. However, the debates which were taking place around maternity increasingly drew in feminists, both as mothers and as midwives. The arguments were not all in the direction of control for women through the use of less technology and a belief in the sanctity of the labour experience. Debates such as that around the availability of epidural analgesia were couched in feminist terms, with the psycho-prophylactic techniques espoused by Dick-Read and latterly by the NCT described as leaving women feeling responsible for their own pain: 'Women now attribute their pain to their own inadequacies and inability to relax … British women are bound by birth conventions which are usually imposed by men. There's no urgency about relieving women of childbirth pain, and indeed apparent pressure to the contrary' *(The Guardian* 12.04.1973). To some women feminism gave them the framework to demand a reconnection with their bodies and with the biological experience of labour. For others it clearly gave them the ammunition to be as far removed as possible from the mess and pain of birth, and delivery in the hours of daylight with an effective epidural were victories rather than failures. There was, therefore, always a plurality of women's voices, which made the work of campaigners, not to mention midwives and doctors, more problematic.

The response of the service

The evidence of women's dissatisfaction with the maternity services built up across the period, partly because there was a growing strand of research which explored their attitude towards pregnancy and birth and the care which they received. This ranged from anecdotal reports built up from letters women wrote about their experiences (Morris 1960) to large-scale quantitative and qualitative research projects (Cartwright 1979; Oakley 1981). As survey data built up, certain issues stood out even as the concentration of maternity services in institutions continued to develop. Antenatal care, and in particular antenatal clinics, were a significant source of concern for women, as was information given by professionals, or the lack thereof. Finally, and fundamentally, women, who were still primarily cared for by midwives, saw the office of midwife in a very different light to those who held it. The evidence suggests that midwives felt themselves to be professionals who had the best interests of women at heart, but whose power and autonomy was challenged across the period by doctors, women and policy makers. Many women, on the other hand, did not view their relationships with midwives as necessarily positive, but saw it as at least potentially demeaning and punitive. This section discusses the response of the maternity service to these elements of debate, together with the changing nature of the relationship between midwives and women across the period.

In 1960 very few women had their partners with them as they laboured. Midwives who worked on the district recalled that sometimes fathers were there, and at other times not, and there is no sense of it being a point of contention or debate either way. Women who delivered in hospital, however, invariably did so alone. This appears to have been a new departure in maternity care since historically women had always been attended by someone, or possibly several people, including friends, relatives and the lay or trained midwife. Even in rushed district midwifery, where the midwife might not arrive until second stage was well advanced, women were rarely completely alone. Hospitals changed all that; they neither had the staff to sit with women, nor the facilities to admit friends or husbands (Christie and Tansey 2001: 57). Women often laboured several to a room, and men did not begin to make an appearance until the physical layout of hospitals began to allow for greater privacy.

The demand for fathers to be allowed to be present during labour and birth was one that was made with increasing confidence by both the NCT and AIMS during the period, and both groups claimed the ultimate credit for the admission of men (Beech and Willington 2007). They were not the only ones; both obstetricians and midwives believed it was their intercession which led to change, but in the teeth of opposition from the other (*The Guardian* 03.02.1971; Christie and Tansey 2001: 58; see Leavitt 2009 for the US perspective). The pressure therefore came from several different angles: groups such as the NCT who felt men should be there as spiritual and emotional support, the NHS because it relieved the pressure on staff, and some doctors and midwives. By 1971 it was reckoned that 10 per cent of men supported their partners through labour and delivery, numbers which were to rocket as attendance came to be increasingly normalised (Barbour 1990). As with every other aspect of maternity care, however, it was not something which all women, never mind all men, wanted:

> My husband was not there which I was quite glad about. I don't like people to see me if I'm in pain as I find it harder to bear. I wouldn't want to see him upset … I'm sorry he missed the actual experience of it, but for me I preferred it that way.
>
> (Devlin 1995: 123)

'Allowing' partners to be present during labour and delivery was one aspect of what came to be described as the humanising of the maternity service. For much of the period, whatever the views of some women, delivery in hospital and the use of technology were regarded by the majority of doctors, midwives and policy makers as non-negotiable. There was a growing acceptance, however, that birth did not have to appear as clinical as it had become, and that changes in the layout of labour rooms or the way clinics were organised were all that were needed to reconcile women to the modern way of birth (Short Report 1980). The evidence for this came from across the period and it would be a mistake to assume, however, that the people who worked in maternity had no conception of the impact of the developing service on the women it cared for, or were cynical about it. One of the first people specifically to discuss the issue was Norman Morris who was Professor of Obstetrics and Gynaecology at Charing Cross Hospital in London, the city where, along with Manchester, the science of obstetrics was seeing its fullest expression. His article drew on letters sent by women to a women's magazine, with tales of impersonal treatment, overcrowded wards and waiting rooms and a casual cruelty by staff. The language he used was powerful, and chimed with that used by campaigners such as Sally Willington: 'The joys, hopes and wonder that the arrival of a new life should bring are spoiled and splintered into loneliness, indignity and despair' (Morris 1960). The hospital system was seen as analogous to that of the factory, and the staff too busy to take notice:

> The midwives at the hospital all seem to have too much on their plate to bother with the odd person who wants to know 'why, where and what'. Whenever I go for treatment it always seems as though I were being put on a conveyer belt and passing through all the different stages – water – blood – examination. There seems to be nothing human in them at times.
>
> (woman quoted in Morris 1960)

The remedy Morris proposed was one which would echo down through the years: to make hospitals more homely, to reduce over-crowding at clinics, and to offer women kindness rather than regimentation (Ministry of Health 1961). The Short Report, published exactly 20 years later made identical points, arguing that midwives with 'warmth' should be employed in sensitive areas such as antenatal clinics, where women were undergoing their first exposure to the maternity services. According to Short, if any women were put off further pregnancies by their experience of the hospital system then that was a failure which had to be remedied through careful handling. Neither Morris, Short nor any of those who debated the issue in the years between necessarily felt that it was the system that was at fault; rather it came down to the way in which it was explained and presented. It was felt that women did not necessarily understand the reasons for the treatments given or the procedures undertaken, and that more explanation would help women not to feel so acted upon. Morris himself pondered the influence of the doctors and midwives who cared for women, arguing that doctors had too little understanding of normal labour, and midwives too little understanding of women and of themselves 'Do midwives who are spinsters past the menopause have to contend with specific emotional complications, which in part are exacerbated by their occupation?' (Morris 1960).

Although he speculated that busyness, emotional distance and a task-driven culture may be a mechanism by which midwives and doctors defended themselves against fear and anxiety, it was to the issue of emotionally unfulfilled midwives that correspondents, wading into the debate engendered by Morris' article, returned:

> ... there is no doubt that so much of the prevailing punitive attitude to pregnant women is the projection onto the prospective mother of the unresolved conflicts concerning sex in the mind of the doctor and the nurse, especially the Senior Hospital Midwife. There is no doubt that many of these women are deeply jealous (often at an unconscious level) of their patients' ability to have children.
>
> (*The Lancet* 1960: 1028)

The attempt to blame the unfulfilled midwives for systemic problems within the maternity services may seem laughable, but the evidence suggests that women's perceptions of those caring for them coloured their experience to a significant extent. To Kitzinger, however, it was more about a state of mind:

> Well many midwives were very authoritarian and thought that it was a sort of games mistress approach almost, that you had to behave yourself as if you were on a hockey field and obeyed the rules, otherwise everything would go to pot.
>
> (Kitzinger interview)

This sentiment was borne out by newspaper articles and letters detailing stories of births under cold and unsympathetic midwives:

> Having been left by myself quite literally for hours I realised I was going to be sick. I rang for a nurse who told me crossly that she would come when she could. As the baby was only within about fifteen minutes of being born I was unable to get up and was sick on the floor. At this the night sister arrived and proceeded to give me a thorough dressing down. This in spite of the fact I had requested nothing since my admittance. Her tirade was cut short owing to my having to be rushed to the labour ward to give birth.
>
> (*The Guardian* 29.07.1960)

The conscious attempt by the service to describe and engage with the issue of 'human relations' suggested significant anxieties by professionals about the way in which birth in particular was coming to be managed. As early as 1962, Myles was reminding midwifery students about the importance of kindliness and care, as well as the provision of hospital rooms with a 'home-like atmosphere'. However, by 1975 Myles had admitted that labour and delivery were akin to a surgical procedure, and the recommendation to provide 'charming pictures' on the walls or a chair in which to knit were gone. Humanising midwifery mattered in the early 1960s because women still exercised agency in their choice of place of birth. By the mid-1970s this had almost disappeared, only to reappear in the early 1980s as consumer demands around pregnancy and birth once again gained momentum.

Relationships between midwives and women were complex, and the stories told about maternity care from each perspective do not always tally. To women, midwives could be cold and bossy, or deeply warm and caring. To the midwife, women could be unnecessarily demanding or laughably ignorant. Both groups used shorthand and concepts of heroic attitudes or behaviour to describe characteristics of the other, in a way that made sense and made a complex and symbiotic relationship more manageable. Storytelling, and the stock figures that go with it, remained part of the experience of maternity for both women and their care givers and even in an age of technology, it was the memory of the human relations which lingered.

However, midwives were part of a system of maternity which was increasingly regarded as discredited by some women, and this impacted on the relationship between mother and midwife. Jean Robinson, who worked for AIMS, remarked in interview that 'midwives sold women down the river' because they were seen as part of the medical establishment, rather than being 'with woman' as the name 'midwife' suggested they should be. She argued that AIMS and other consumer groups 'were hampered not just by the arrogance of the medical profession and their entrenched and undeniable power, but by the weakness of the midwives ... they are no fighters and they do not think strategically.'

The situation was complicated by the fact that there was also a pride among midwives that they were professionals and they did know best. One midwife who worked in Manchester in the 1970s felt that many women had their expectations of pregnancy and birth raised by consumer groups, and that any recourse to technology or assistance was seen by women as constituting 'failure' which midwives then had to deal with (Stella interview). There was also pride among midwives who worked in rural communities that they knew 'their' women well, and the relationship was an individual one rather than needing to be mediated through the language of 'control' or 'rights' (Doris interview).

One midwife, Jenny, who worked in Nottingham in the 1970s and 1980s, said that she felt relationships between women and midwives were good in the 1970s because 'They didn't have the expectations that they have now, and trusted you I think probably.' Another midwife reflected that in many ways this relationship could itself be dangerous:

Well my experience over the years is that midwives are wonderful at relating to women, and truthfully they can sell them anything, and this is what they did and actually continued to do, really, to a large degree. You have a wonderful rapport with the women you care for and if you feel fairly confident that you're doing the right thing, then the women will put their trust in you and go with the flow. So it wasn't sold as anything spectacular, it was just the way to go that you will be induced and this'll be how it happens.

(Jane interview)

The move from 'patient' to 'consumer' affected midwives because they felt their professional status was being eroded. Jenny described the impact that this had on their work and on their professional standing: 'I think the women's and families' expectations were far greater than we could ever provide.' This she attributed to government policy and to the demands of women, but also the squeeze between expectations and the ability of the service to cope. This included not just lack of staff and equipment, but lack of respect by doctors, particularly in the large teaching hospitals, for the work that midwives did. Jenny felt midwives were regarded as pliable handmaidens both by doctors and increasingly by some women; and that their demands could be incompatible.

Within the rhetoric of urban consumer groups there was no attempt to include the voices or needs of non-middle-class members of the community such as women from low-income families, refugees, teenage mothers or single mothers. Mavis Kirkham, who worked as a hospital midwife in Sheffield in the 1970s, described consciously deploying 'nice middle class' couples to pioneer partners being present in theatre for elective Caesareans, because they would be least threatening to doctors and most able to articulate their belief in their rights. Within her practice, she spoke of 'misfits' coming together; not just midwives who did not fit the system but women as well, who found and supported each other. In many ways these were still an elite self-selected group; women who were articulate and well read and confident enough to demand a particular kind of care. Kirkham suggested that change came incrementally, through individuals attending antenatal classes, or booking with a certain community midwife, but it is debatable how far it impacted on the experiences which the majority of women had of maternity care. In contrast, Oakley's work on the experience of first-time pregnancy and motherhood, conducted between 1975 and 1976, demonstrates that women continued to be accepting of the system as it was (Oakley 1981). This was not to say they were always happy with it, but they had no language for criticising the system, and no sense that they could change it. These were ordinary women living in an urban environment; not people with the confidence to write to MPs or the money to buy into a philosophy such as natural birth.

A thread which has run through the history of midwifery is the inability of midwives to support each other, either on an individual basis or in support of wider professional issues. Caroline Flint, an independent midwife and no stranger to controversy, described midwifery as 'a very punitive profession' (Christie and Tansey 2001: 32) and this is often how it appeared to members, but also to women.

However, campaigners accepted that a supportive midwife could ameliorate many of the traumas associated with birth in the 1970s (Jean Robinson interview). Robinson also expressed the belief that these midwives were disappearing:

> We were going to lose, within the folklore of women and within the training of midwives and doctors, what normal birth was. And that the experience of normal birth came from all these women who had been employed by local authorities, who'd gone round on their little bicycles, been very poorly paid, worked God knows awful hours but had the knowledge of the range of normal and this individual one-to-one care.
>
> (Jean Robinson interview)

The language used is in itself quite paternalistic, and the image it draws is that of the midwife who approached her career as if it was a calling and whose work was her life. It did not, as Robinson tacitly accepted, represent a way of life to which many midwives would wish to return.

The *Perinatal Mortality Survey*, gave a powerful, if as it turned out, somewhat erroneous view of the relative safety of different places of birth, and also an insight into the work of midwives as the 1950s shaded into the 1960s, and provides a snap-shot of patterns of care. Some of the figures belie the wider arguments about types of birth and levels of intervention, demonstrating that whatever doctors believed about their power and influence, it was midwives who continued to provide the majority of care and to deliver the vast majority of babies. Midwives and their supervised pupils delivered around 85 per cent of babies in both domiciliary and hospital settings, and in over 70 per cent of cases a midwife was the senior professional present during labour and delivery. Maureen, who worked as a district midwife in the 1960s, described the routine of care in ways which had not changed much in 50 years:

> Well, we'd make sure that labour was established and it usually was with them. Then we would prepare her for delivery and prepare the bed, and then just make sure it was warm … they had no central heating so we had to make sure, especially in the winter times, that we had heating in there, just make sure we'd got some hot water, and just keep an eye on the blood pressure, contractions and dilation and this sort of thing as labour progressed, and dad used to come up with cups of tea. Not often the husband was there – he didn't often stay in those days … They were around usually and often the next door neighbour was there or the mother was there …
>
> (Maureen interview)

Antenatal education was increasingly offered, and included relaxation and breathing, which midwives felt made a difference to the way in which women experienced labour (Maureen interview; Barbara interview). However, district midwives still remembered themselves as having had the time to be with women in labour and it was this relationship rather than the application of particular techniques, which many – both midwives and women – saw as key to their ability to cope. This was reinforced by postnatal visiting, which although officially prescriptive, clearly gave many midwives the opportunity to offer as much, or as little, as the mother and her family seemed to need:

> ... we went in twice a day for three days and then once a day up until I think the 14th day, but the 11th and 13th day we didn't go, unless there was something that made us go. And I mean if at three days, we felt this mum needs more than one visit a day, we would still visit the two times, the twice a day.
>
> (Maureen interview)

The link between the midwife and her community was, however, changed beyond recognition with the 1974 Health Act. This ushered in the break-up of the tripartite system of maternity care, which had been urged as far back as the Guillebaud Report, and most recently by the Peel Report. Broadly, the change saw the final triumph of acute medicine with the dismantling of the apparatus of local authority care and the position of the Medical Officer of Health. For midwifery specifically, it meant the first significant change to the organisation of the service since the 1936 Midwives Act, with all midwives, whether community or hospital based, now coming under the umbrella of the acute services. The MoH for Nottingham had noted the writing on the wall in 1969:

> With the advent of the GP obstetrician and the recommendation that all confinements should take place in hospital and early return home, the Local Authority has no further part to play in the care of expectant mothers. Its obligation to provide a midwifery service has become obsolete.
>
> (*MoH Report Nottingham* 1969: 40)

For many women the change was not significant, but for many midwives it had huge consequences. Julia Allison described the break-up of the local authority-led midwifery service as having a very negative effect on many district midwives because it eroded their autonomy, and was the final nail in the coffin of any concerted attempt to provide a domiciliary midwifery service (Julia Allison interview). For some midwives the change clearly came as a relief as it reduced their need to be available for duty at all times of day and night, and allowed midwifery to assume the status of work rather than of some all-encompassing calling. For others, however, it destroyed everything they believed about their work (Julia Allison interview). One GP described the impact that this had on the district midwife with whom he worked:

> The parting of the ways between myself and Ann came about because she couldn't swallow this anymore, she couldn't see herself just as an antenatal and postnatal nurse. She was too acutely involved with her skills as an accoucheur for her to be able to accept it. It is very difficult indeed to give up skills that you are capable of exercising because there has been a change in policy. She saw her role as a professional being diminished.
>
> (Aspinall et al. 1997)

By 1980 there was a clear sense that midwifery was teetering on the brink of extinction, not for legal reasons, but partly through a lack of practitioners and partly as a result of the de-skilling and over-work evident in both community and hospital midwifery (Robinson 1980). Sheila Kitzinger was among those who argued that 'with the modern emphasis on technology, our midwives are being increasingly downgraded and treated more and more like obstetric nurses in the United States rather than as professionals in their own right' (*The Times* 13.05.1980). She linked the re-skilling of midwives back to the need to develop alternative models of care, particularly those based on domiciliary work. Needless to say, this brought a thunderous response from some doctors, with one Fellow of RCOG suggesting that 'Midwifery is too important to be left exclusively to midwives' and that even the most experienced midwife would not be capable of coping with the manifold dangers of home birth (*The Times* 21.05.1980). Meanwhile Sarah Robinson, who was exploring the role of the midwife for a DHSS-funded research project, found that the style and pace of work was causing not just practical problems for midwives, but emotional and professional ones too:

> Not enough time for midwives to fulfil their duties as they want to. Notable especially on labour ward where too few midwives can lead to care which lacks continuity, abnormalities of labour may be missed until more serious, dissatisfied staff and patients.
>
> (midwife quoted in Robinson 1980: 19)

This impacted significantly on how midwives felt about their work:

> I can't begin to explain adequately: we frequently miss meal breaks. We are rushing from patient to patient in labour trying to cope. Because of the pressure and nature of the work there is no job satisfaction, and most midwives feel exploited and overworked, consequently they leave to do other jobs which exacerbates the situation.
>
> (midwife quoted in Robinson 1980: 23)

Midwives were as attuned to a sense of heroics as were doctors. Chloe Fisher, a midwife who worked initially on the district in Oxfordshire, commented that

'At the time we still worked as partners, midwives, and so we worked crazy hours and we were on-call 24 hours and I'm sure that we were unsafe sometimes, but thank goodness nothing awful happened to me' (Christie and Tansey 2001: 28). This almost macho attitude seems at odds with the image of the caring mid-wife, but chimed with many midwives' views of themselves as central to the maternity service. Although it suited some midwives, there was however a sense that not only was it not safe, it limited the numbers of women who would choose midwifery as a career. In 1965 an article in the *Midwives Chronicle* drew attention to the physical and mental strain under which mid-wives were working, and questioned its ethical basis; this was echoed 15 years later by the midwives who responded to Robinson's survey (1980).

Looking back, midwives who worked through the period demonstrate almost a sense of shock that they were unable to halt the developments taking place, despite believing that they did not have the professional or political power to have an impact. More pertinently than that, however, it was hard to recognise the broader landscape of change when caught up in the minutiae of work; a midwife who worked through the period commented that:

> Once women went into hospital and booked under obstetricians, the midwifery profession started to decline. It was very easy with hindsight to see that. My generation of midwives has to bear the responsibility for it but at the time we were just too busy getting on with our job to notice the erosion of our role.
>
> (Christie and Tansey 2001: 14)

This was echoed by Doris who worked in Lincolnshire in the 1960s and 1970s, and commented that it was only by looking back that the magnitude of the changes and the impact that this had on both midwives and women became evident.

Jean Robinson described midwives as being 'powerless' and suggested that they caved into hospital pressures (interview). For this she blamed midwifery organisations, arguing that midwives were vital to the service and should have been able 'to get the moon for themselves and their members'. However, she did admit that for articulate middle-class lay campaigners, it was easy to make a fuss, because they did not put their jobs on the line with every protest:

> We could rant and rave and publish stuff or do press releases or broadcast, but it wasn't our job, our mortgage, our food on the table, our career on the line. It's the people trying to fight on the inside and often being picked off one by one because they weren't supported by their colleagues, they're the ones who are the courageous ones.
>
> (Jean Robinson interview)

However, just as the feminist and consumer movements impacted on women, they changed the terms of the debate about their working lives for some midwives. There were groups of midwives who were instrumental in developing a different discourse and in working alongside women, in particular the Association of Radical Midwives (ARM) which was formed in 1976 by a group of student midwives, who themselves felt oppressed by the system under which they worked.

The independent midwife Caroline Flint described ARM as having a 'huge impact' on midwifery, although evidence from rank and file midwives who worked during this period throws up no memories of the organisation, except amongst its committed membership. For those who were involved, however, its influence was significant, and reflected a developing feminist awareness as much as a midwifery one:

> But those meetings were wonderful and we learned all sorts of things. It was also, of course, the feminist women's health movement, self-examination, all these things were at their peak. So we peered at each other's cervixes, cannulated each other and we learnt all these things, like you do.
>
> (Mavis Kirkham interview)

Kirkham admitted that the group never had the numbers or the power to challenge the prevailing system on a grand scale. Rather she described ARM as a place of support for midwives who felt, as she described it, like 'refugees from the system'. In terms of political influence, however, their efforts were dismissed by some of the consumer campaigners; Kitzinger argued that they were not a major influence on changes in maternity care (interview).

Conclusion

The story of the period between 1960 and 1980 was that of the decisive move of birth from home to hospital. This had, however, been foreshadowed since the inter-war period and did not represent a break in experience but rather a move along the continuum towards the industrialisation and regulation of pregnancy and birth. No one group was controlling the development, but rather it was as a result of a multiplicity of factors and voices. Middle-class women clamoured for the right to have their babies in hospital, but did not necessarily like what they found when they got there. There was a growing sense among some women that their control over the experience of birth was being eroded by the emphasis on physical risk, on time limits and on statistical measurements of safety and success. Similarly some midwives, who prided themselves on their status as professionals, embraced technology, although others felt their role was being eroded not just by technology and policy but by the demands and expectations of women. All those concerned with birth, whether feminists who wanted a sense of control over their biology, doctors who believed that ultrasound or induction could reduce the risks of pregnancy, or midwives who wanted to control their working lives, struggled with the basic messiness and unpredictability of pregnancy and birth. It was not amenable to strictly imposed time limits, and predicting the limits of risk and safety were fraught with difficulty, particularly as relatively easily measured and understood indices such as maternal mortality receded almost to vanishing point. All of those involved in the experience of maternity appear to have struggled to hear and understand each other, not surprisingly, given that there was not, in reality, just one story to be told; some women wanted high technology hospital births, some wanted the opposite, some just wanted to get it over with and move into motherhood. Similarly some midwives and GPs cherished their domiciliary intra-partum role, others were happy to focus their skills on ante- and postnatal care. The next chapter will consider how these different groups came together in pursuit of the reframing of maternity care which saw the middle-class view emerge, at least superficially, triumphant.

6   1981–2002

Introduction

This chapter covers a period when the tone of the wider social debate around childbirth changed dramatically. It is bisected by the *Changing Childbirth* Report of 1993 written by a government-appointed 'Expert Maternity Group', which was created as a result of the Report of the Health Select Committee published in 1992 (known as the 'Winterton Report'). *Changing Childbirth* has been credited with catalysing debate around care in pregnancy and during birth, and in revolutionising even the language used to frame it. In many ways, however, *Changing Childbirth* was not the break with the past that it at first appears and, as with previous government reports, it simply codified developments which were already underway. However, it was widely perceived at the time as being of seminal importance. This chapter will consider the reasons behind this and the legacy left by the Report. As well as altering the tone of the national discourse around birth, *Changing Childbirth* also impacted on the way in which midwifery viewed itself. By the late 1980s the profession – although there were debates as to whether it could even be described as such – was feeling increasingly beleaguered. It seemed beset on one side by the demands of high-technology obstetric care and on the other by the growing numbers of women articulating their demands for a particular type of care. The impact of *Changing Childbirth* on home birth or choice was probably, ultimately, more symbolic than real, but it did restore midwives to what they saw as their rightful place in the hierarchy of the maternity care system by making explicit that they were the guardians of 'normality'.

This chapter will, therefore, critically present the development and results of the *Changing Childbirth* Report on the wider landscape of maternity care. Beyond these confines it will also explore the continued development of a plurality of voices in maternity; whether through the NCT, the Active Birth movement, or the campaigns to support those who stood outside the mainstream, including obstetrician Wendy Savage. These voices, emboldened by the language of *Changing Childbirth*, added to the clamour for a new beginning in maternity. The development of midwifery-led care, renewed (if patchy) support for home birth, and a growing emphasis on the public health role of the midwife saw a quickening pace in the development of midwifery itself. This chapter will, however, focus on a new professional project for midwives as they sought to engage with research and education in order to cement their role at the centre of maternity.

Demonstrating for change

One of the most vocal proponents for change in the culture of birth in the early 1980s was Janet Balaskas who developed what she coined the 'Active Birth Movement' (a play on the idea of 'active management of birth' which was heavily promoted in hospitals at the time). Following the managed birth of her first child, Balaskas joined the NCT and learned to be an antenatal teacher under Sheila Kitzinger. She eventually moved into teaching yoga, modified for pregnancy and birth, and together with Michel Odent (a French obstetrician) was one of the first advocates of the use of water immersion for labour and birth (Balaskas 1991; Balaskas and Gordon 1992). She developed a philosophy around birth which took in concepts of feminism, spirituality and psychology, particularly in relation to bonding. Balaskas described the development of her work with reference to her own personal experiences of pregnancy and birth, but also to the stories she heard from other women. These discourses echoed ideas about midwifery knowledge, with midwives who trained and worked in the mid-century described as being distilled from a mixture of lived experience and what might be described as storytelling with a purpose. Balaskas described her use of research evidence to back up her work, but her beliefs clearly came before the research. Some of her ideas, particularly around the efficacy of mobility and upright positions for labour and birth, were beginning to find currency in other areas. In 1978 a small study had appeared in the *BMJ* which reported that labour was shorter in women who were ambulant (Flynn et al. 1978); this followed a handful of earlier studies. Balaskas described the development of her understanding in relation to the new orthodoxy of NCT teaching:

> And then when I started sitting in on my first NCT classes back in those days as part of the training, I noticed that at the reunion sessions, very few women had achieved a natural birth, although most of them were hoping for one, in actual fact, the results weren't that great. This was partly because the environment where they had to give birth was so inhibitory of a normal, natural labour.
>
> (Janet Balaskas interview)

This was an indication of the cultural struggles which were still occurring, and which were highlighted when Balaskas left the NCT because it felt her work was, at that time, unproven (Balaskas interview; Kitzinger interview). As will be seen in relation to *Changing Childbirth*, the NCT was very adept at working the system from within, whereas Balaskas was more iconoclastic in her approach. Even within this, however, she was constrained by prevailing beliefs; the publishers of her first book insisted that it was first read by an obstetrician for approval. For her the defining point was, however, the demonstration organised in support of the use of active birth at the Royal Free Hospital in London:

> ... some of the more conventional consultants, including the Head of the Department, and some of the midwives thought this was absolutely unsafe, animal behaviour; if you got on all fours, you'd have an air embolism, this was very dangerous. And they put out an edict that women shouldn't be allowed to do all this nonsense, resulting in an incidence once where an American woman who was there having her baby was almost physically forced up off all fours or made to sign a disclaimer when she was in transition, and she threw a jug of water at a midwife. So these kind of things happened. But I thought no, this is wrong. The battle isn't in the labour room, the battle has to be outside the labour room.
>
> (Janet Balaskas interview)

The resulting 'Birth Rights Rally' was supported not just by the NCT and AIMS but by the RCM, and drew several thousand protesters who listened to speeches by Odent, Kitzinger and the newsreader Anna Ford as well as Balaskas herself (Balaskas interview; *The Times* 05.04.1982). One of the memories shared by both Balaskas and Kitzinger is of the police who were guiding the demonstration wanting to tell their own stories of labour and birth and what they and their partners had experienced. The debate around birth developed with a series of Active Birth Conferences organised by Balaskas in the early 1980s and attended by up to 3,000 people each time. She argued that 'So the activism that I've done has been really involved in drawing pioneers together and presenting that to the public' (interview). The growing willingness of at least some groups of women to protest and demonstrate showed a development in the tactics of engagement with policy makers and professionals which had traditionally been espoused by the NCT and AIMS. Balaskas claimed that the new 'grass-roots' style of activism was more effective than persuading professionals, although she also accepted that the older groups began to take on board ideas around active or water birth. Underneath this activity there was, however, a belief that such ideas continued to be the preserve of the middle classes, a charge that Balaskas did not dispute. In a piece in *The Times* (15.10.1982) the author, Penny Perrick, commented that:

> There was a danger, I thought, that the active birth movement might become a monument to privilege, confined to middle class and articulate women whose 'right to choose' is seldom threatened since they can afford to pay for their preference. A woman who has the time and money to attend active birth classes and who can pick a consultant whose ideas

coincide with their own is a different case from the woman whose GP just hands her over to the nearest maternity hospital.

This was a charge that Balaskas did not attempt to refute. Instead she suggested, in the same article, that 'Women like us can help effect changes for other women who don't have our opportunities.' Durward and Evans (1990) suggested that by the early 1980s other groups were beginning to appear which gave voice to different sectors of society, particularly those underrepresented in traditional groups such as ethnic minority women. However, although groups such as The Tower Hamlets Maternity Services Liaison Scheme were successful at a grass-roots level, they did not have the political power that middle-class campaigners were able to muster.

Beyond the debates between consumers, however, was the continued thread of the debates around birth by and between professionals. Midwives attended Balaskas' rally and conferences, and there is evidence that they began to incorporate ideas of active birth into practice (Mavis interview). The official seal of approval came, however, when *Mayes' Midwifery* textbook, which had made no mention of the issue in its 1984 edition, devoted a section in its 1988 edition to the issue of squatting in labour. As Sweet commented in her preface, however, it was important not to let things go too far:

> Many [parents] desire natural childbirth and require more information, more autonomy and less intervention in this major event in their lives. In this new edition I have attempted to strike a balance between the needs and demands of parents and the major scientific and technological advances which, provided they are used wisely and selectively, can be of great benefit to childbearing women and their babies.
>
> (Sweet 1988: ix)

Despite this veiled attempt at support for consumer wishes, the central issues for campaigners such as Balaskas was still around the power of doctors; the Birth Rights rally was organised in support of Yehudi Gordon, an obstetrician at the Royal Free Hospital who championed active birth and was suspended from practice for doing so. The other demonstrations seen in London around the issue of birth in the early 1980s occurred in support of another consultant, also suspended as a result of her practice: Wendy Savage. Savage's case became a *cause célèbre* after she was suspended for alleged professional incompetence, following 25 years working in medicine. The case against centred around her unwillingness to intervene in labour in what she regarded as an unnecessary fashion, and boiled down to a professional dispute between obstetricians over the clinical management of labour, particularly complex labour. Just as Balaskas had done over the dispute with the Royal Free Hospital, Savage and her supporters were able to harness the power of the ever more confident consumer groups such as the NCT to fight their cause. This dispute did not take place in the leafy environs of Hampstead, however, but the poor working-class and ethically diverse East End of London (Savage 1988). For all the demonstrations, rallies and fund raising, however, and for all Savage's support for midwifery practice, the issue was around consultant hegemony. Savage, whose feminism was significant to her, believed in including women in decision making around labour, and was concerned at the level of medicalisation developing around obstetric practice (*The Times* 12.06.1985). Her opponents believed equally strongly in the power and the responsibility of the consultant to decide on plans of care and interventions. The case demonstrated the developing strength of women's voices, still primarily centred around seasoned campaigners such as Kitzinger. It was also, in some ways, a final hurrah for the power of the GP in obstetrics. Although their practice in midwifery had been largely emasculated, it was GPs who supported Savage most vociferously, and she in turn paid tribute to their skill and knowledge of their patients as 'family doctors'. The big success for consumer groups and radical obstetricians and midwives alike had to wait, however, until the final decade of the century.

Changing childbirth

The development, publication and subsequent trajectory of the *Changing Childbirth* Report has to be seen within the wider context of debate around health in this period. The National Health Service (NHS) had been in existence for over 30 years by 1980; long enough for its first generation of children to grow into parenthood themselves. Despite all the beliefs and the promises, however, equality of health in particular seemed to be as far away as it had been in the 1930s. The *Black Report* on health inequalities which was published in 1980, and its successor the *Health Divide*, which appeared eight years later (Townsend et al. 1992), drew attention to some of the broad social factors which they suggested helped to determine differential risks of ill-health and life span. Both Reports argued, much to the chagrin of political leaders at the time, that health inequalities had in fact risen since the inception of the NHS. Even in areas where total mortality had fallen – including maternal mortality – the relative differences between classes remained or even increased. This fed into a wider debate about what actually constituted health, and whether it was appropriate to focus on a narrow medical definition, or whether the influence of wider social issues was so great that they had to be viewed as part of the equation (Berridge et al. 2006). In talking of the money spent on the NHS successive governments tended to favour the narrower definition, and indeed the development of the NHS, with its focus on hospitals, beds, consultants and cures, was predicated on this belief. Maternity services, an integral part of the NHS behemoth, in many respects followed the prevailing debate; particularly evinced in the 1974 reorganisation which lumped together all maternity services under the umbrella of the acute sector.

Despite this, maternity was one of the first areas which saw a challenge both to the power of the acute sector and the hegemony of reductive measures of success including maternal or perinatal mortality. However, the impetus for the debate did not come from policy makers or from practitioners, but from women's groups and from researchers outside the service (Berridge et al. 2006: 69). As early as ten years after the founding of the NHS, a debate was developing around the importance of psychological, as opposed simply to physical indicators of a successful maternity experience (Morris 1960). These hard to quantify measures of mental well-being or enhanced self-esteem had, it was argued, as much impact on health and perceptions of health, as did measures of lives saved or lost. When infant and maternal mortality remained higher, in relative and absolute terms, among lower social groups the challenge was, however, to bring this reframed debate down to the reach of all (Acheson Report 1988). It was doctors in particular who argued that it was all very well for the privileged middle classes to demand emotional satisfaction from the business of childbirth; what remained problematic was to include all sectors of society. With growing perceptions of the existence of an 'underclass' who did not share wider social norms, it became an increasing challenge for policy makers and practitioners to reach out to and care for this minority at a time when the terms of the debate appeared to be set by the articulate middle classes. The concept of an underclass became enshrined in the language of 'social exclusion' which developed over this period and, within the maternity services, came to encompass a variety of 'problem' areas including teenagers, drug users, ethnic minorities, the homeless and refugees (see for example Social Exclusion Unit 1999). The language used suggested that these were groups who needed to be helped and encouraged to take a particular view of such issues as antenatal care or infant rearing. The unspoken implication was that there was a right way and a wrong way to approach maternity as an individual and that the government and health agencies and professionals would encourage the right way; this was made clear by the recommendations of the Acheson Report (1988) which emphasised individual measures to tackle health inequality such as smoking cessation, diet, or breastfeeding support. 'Health promotion', a concept developed particularly through the World Health Organization, was enthusiastically taken up by public health officials and by policy makers (Berridge et al. 2006). It has been suggested that maternity-based consumer groups such as the NCT had a significant impact on the re-casting of public health generally, in the years following 1974 and the break-up of the role of the local MoH (Moscucci in Berridge et al. 2006: 68). Running underneath all these debates, there was, however, an almost plaintive sense of confusion that the welfare state in general and the NHS in particular had not succeeded in making health inequalities disappear and had not managed, in health terms, to make everyone middle class.

Although vilified by policy makers at the time, both the *Black Report* and the *Health Divide* in suggesting wider causality for health problems across society, paradoxically both broadened and polarised the debate.

Elements of the maternity services did pick up on the challenges laid down by the *Black Report*, with efforts, for example, to decentralise antenatal clinics in order to make them more accessible to women without transport. There was a whole raft of such measures promulgated in the 1980s (Dowling 1984). Efforts were made to reach out to those sections of society perceived to be on the wrong side of the 'health divide'. It could be argued, ironically, that it was the creation of a centralised acute-based maternity service which had exacerbated any problems in the first place by depersonalising care. Doris felt that the relationship she had with 'her' women in the late 1960s allowed her to identify and support women with problems quickly and unobtrusively:

> If you had a postnatal depression ... because we were on very good terms with the Health Visitor, we could share visits because it can get very ... we had some very bad ones, as they do today but the difference was we probably picked them up because we were in more. I had someone that took slug pellets and I had an awful job to get her admitted with a GP. Before he would admit her, we were going backwards and forwards, in every day. I've spoken to her many times since and she said she felt she had to do it to [herself] or [she]'d have done something to the baby. But you see you did pick them up ... so we all knew in some ways where to expect the problems because it's often the house proud.
>
> (Doris interview)

Some of the issues surrounding maternity moved to the political centre stage with the publication of *Changing Childbirth* which was widely disseminated and reported with its ideas and recommendations discussed in lay circles and newspapers as well as in professional journals. At the heart of the Report was what appeared to be a revolutionary change in the way that pregnancy and childbirth were characterised. It followed the lead of the Winterton Report which stated categorically, and given previous official pronouncements, quite startlingly, that:

> On the basis of what we have heard, this Committee must draw the conclusion that the policy of encouraging all women to give birth in hospital cannot be justified on the grounds of safety ... Given the absence of conclusive evidence, it is no longer acceptable that the pattern of maternity care provision should be driven by presumptions about the applicability of a medical model of care based on unproven assertions.
>
> (Winterton Report 1992: xii)

Throughout *Changing Childbirth* it was reiterated that pregnancy and birth were natural physiological events, rather than pathologically based emergencies, and that the medical model of care was not appropriate to the majority of maternity service users. Certainly in so far as the Report was developed, the language it used of choice and control for women, and the development of women-centred care reflected a different approach to evidence gathering. Although members of groups such as the NCT had been called to give evidence to Government Committees as far back as the Cranbrook Report of 1959, *Changing Childbirth* was the first example of the power of consumer groups in setting the maternity agenda. The President of the NCT, Eileen Hutton, sat on the Committee as an expert, and surveys were conducted as part of the work of the group to explore the views of service users. This meant that, unlike in previous national reports where the views of obstetricians in particular held sway, the psycho-social aspects of maternity care were fore-grounded. This had two vital knock-on effects. The first, and very striking, was the refusal of the Report to engage in the relative safety or otherwise of home or hospital birth. *Changing Childbirth* suggested that wherever women felt safest was probably where they were safest. Beyond that, however, it did not comment on what was a vociferous and hard-fought battle between the two factions. The second key aspect of the concentration on psycho-social aspects was the foregrounding of the role of the midwife. This historically vilified and feted figure was henceforth to be characterised as the lead pro-fessional in normal pregnancy, birth and the puerperium. This was a powerful and categorical statement which was to resonate throughout midwifery.

The Report did actually make clear that it was in many ways drawing attention to, and applauding changes that were already occurring in the maternity services, particularly around team working and communication. By the early 1990s, 40 per cent of maternity units in England had experimented with different forms of team midwifery in order to address issues of poor continuity of care for women. As well as being consumer driven, some of these developments drew on wider management debates in nursing in parti-cular about patient-centred care. Research tended to highlight the mechan-istic, and from the patient's point of view, deleterious, nature of process- or task-driven care. It was argued that routines such as doing all patient obser-vations at a set time suited the factory nature of hospital, allowing a large number of patients to be 'processed' in a short space of time by relatively few staff. What got lost, however, was the human aspect of nursing care, together with missed opportunities to diagnose and treat as a result of fragmented and partial care. This issue was reflected in debates in nursing about how best to provide individualised patient-centred care (Roper et al. 1990). Many of the debates in maternity about the impersonality of care, which reached back to the early 1960s and *Human Relations in Obstetrics* (1961), were not therefore unique to the service and nor were their solutions unique to *Changing Childbirth*.

The *Changing Childbirth* Report generated a significant amount of pub-licity and debate. To understand the reasons for this it is useful briefly to compare the language and style of the Report with that of its predecessors, the three linked publications of the Maternity Services Advisory Committee. These Reports, which separately covered antenatal, intra-partum and postnatal care, were ordered by the government in the wake of the Short Report of 1980 (discussed in the previous chapter) and relied on evidence already collected as well as its belief in its own expertise. To this end the Committee claimed that its membership of doctors and midwives enabled it to produce 'authoritative guidelines' which would be taken up by all practitioners. This meant that statements so often repeated through government and other official or quasi-official reports were made again without examination. The beliefs that birth should take place in hospital and that there was a direct correlation between antenatal care and reduced maternal and perinatal death rates were presented without debate. This was despite the growing discomfort voiced by Tew (1995) and others about the reliability of the links between safety and medical care. As far as official policy was concerned little had changed since the *Perinatal Mortality Survey* of 1963 (Butler and Bonham).

In other ways, however, the Reports of the Maternity Services Advisory Committee did foreshadow at least the language that was later to be used by *Changing Childbirth*. In discussing antenatal care it was commented that:

> The first visit should provide an opportunity for the woman to meet members of the health care team with whom she will be in contact throughout her pregnancy. The woman should leave the clinic feeling that she has been treated as a responsible partner who can play an important part in what lies ahead, and whose wishes will be respected. She should be quite clear about all the services available to her and how to obtain them ...
>
> (Maternity Services Advisory Committee, Part 1 1982: 8)

This does not necessarily promote, or even suggest, choice, but it does offer a sense of dialogue between women and health professionals. Beyond this the Reports recommended both that the full range of midwives' skills should be utilised more effectively by the service and that issues of public health should be foregrounded. From the point of view of the midwifery service, particularly the community team, this meant an emphasis on personal issues of public health such as smoking, diet and infant feeding. There was no discussion of midwives as lead professionals in any aspect of maternity care, but rather their status as a member of the 'team' was reiterated. In general the trio of Reports did not philosophise about maternity care but were operational in their approach to trying to marry beliefs about safety, based on the belief that pregnancy and birth were only normal in retrospect, with at least an acknowledgement of the human relations aspect of the service. Even at this point, in the early 1980s, it is clear that the demands of women were being incorporated into the service at least at some levels. During birth, for example, the report stated that:

> During delivery, the mother should adopt the position which she feels is most comfortable and effective, provided this allows the safe birth of her baby. The midwife or doctor attending her should endeavour to adapt to the position the mother wishes to take.
>
> (Maternity Services Advisory Committee, Part 2 1984: 10)

Clearly this statement was attempting to have it both ways in arguing that the woman should have control over her birth, but offering it back to the health professional under the guise of safety. In fact ARM, through its journal *Midwifery Matters* (1985), welcomed the Report.

Despite the 'definitive' statement of policy and of the care which should be offered which the reports put forward, the 1980s demonstrated a level of anxious debate amongst professionals, to compliment the insistent ones of consumer groups, about the tenor and direction of the maternity services. The publication *Pregnancy Care in the 1980s* (Zander and Chamberlain 1984), a collection of essays and discussions by leading obstetricians, epidemiologists, statisticians, consumers and even the odd midwife, highlighted many of the emerging debates and drew attention not only to disagreements between professionals about the best models of care, but also to the dissonance between what they felt the maternity services offered and what women seemed to be suggesting that they were experiencing. It clearly felt at times to some health professionals that their best efforts to provide a maternity service were almost wilfully misconstrued by service users. The provision of ultrasound scanning was one such issue; whilst some consumer groups argued that it was under-researched technology as far as safety was concerned, and its use should be proscribed, some doctors felt foetal images were what women wanted and needed, not least in order to bond with their babies (Beech and Robinson 1996; Tansey and Christie 2000). Medicine was therefore presented as a passive tool, subject entirely to the demands of women. As Jean Robinson, one of those who were concerned about the use of ultrasound, herself commented (interview) the topic was a fraught one for campaigners against the blanket use of technology because it was generally popular with women, in a way that induction of labour was not. Debates around the relative safety of places and types of birth were closely argued. There is a powerful sense in these essays that doctors in particular, both obstetricians and a committed rump of GPs (including Luke Zander who co-edited the collection) felt that they were doing the right thing, and were left casting around for reasons why women might be so severe about their efforts. The thread running through many of the discussions in the book was that the system was broadly right, particularly now that the worst excesses of the induction of labour era of the 1970s had gone. What was wrong was the communication between services and women. Chapters in *Pregnancy Care for the 1980s* therefore focused on why women failed to access antenatal care, or how to make hospital labour wards more attractive with the development of wall-papered birth rooms. There is very much a sense of wounded professional sensibilities on show, with contributions from midwives in particular quite plaintive in their calls for more responsibility and regard. There is also a feeling that those involved in the maternity services were grasping for consensus, particularly around the issues of safety, risk and resource allocation.

Beyond the strictures of the Maternity Services Advisory Committee Reports and the soul searching of health professionals about the future of maternity care, there was another wider strand of national debate which fed directly into the language and philosophy of the *Changing Childbirth* Report. Towards the end of the 1980s a national survey manual was published with the aim of giving District Health Authorities and others a template with which to measure 'consumer' views of the maternity services. The concept of the 'patient' as 'consumer' was one which developed across the period in maternity, led by groups such as the NCT who saw themselves as a consumer voice. The language was not, however, restricted to maternity. Government-led changes in the way that the NHS was run, with the development of 'internal markets' and the designation of health services as 'providers' of care, meant that patients across the spectrum were increasingly seen as 'consumers'. This development of language was in many ways based on prevailing political ideologies, but the earlier identification of groups such as the NCT or the Patients Association under Jean Robinson, of themselves as consumers of care – even if that word was not explicitly used – meant that the concept had currency which reached back to the 1970s at least. Government initiatives such as the *Patient's Charter* (1991) were designed to codify the relationship between consumers and providers of health care. The document spoke of patients' 'rights' although there was no legal redress offered if these were not met (Klein 1995). The Charter, which covered the maternity services, suggested that women should know the name of their midwife, and have any tests undertaken explained to them. In many ways this was an indictment of the system of care which had prevailed, whereby women had screening or medication they knew nothing about and to which they had not consented. The Charter made no mention of options of place; the assumption being, even as the *Changing Childbirth* Report was making headlines, that birth would take place in hospital. Even the, arguably anodyne, statement of intent offered by the Charter drew the fire of some professionals. In *Midwifery Matters*, one writer felt the offer of a 'named midwife' was insulting to midwives who all gave excellent care. This was disputed by a mother who complained in the next issue that named midwives, and the sense of personal care and responsibility which that entailed, were in fact exactly what women wanted. Despite *Changing Childbirth*, debate over professional hegemony and consumer influence continued to rage.

Researchers and students have continued to invoke the legacy and language of *Changing Childbirth* and its echoes can be seen in succeeding national reports such as *Maternity Matters* (2007). For consumer groups and for midwives' organisations the Report was, even at the time, talismanic. It did not essentially say anything which was not already being mooted by other groups and other reports (Ball et al. 1992; NHS Management Executive 1993). What made it resonate, however, was the clear and unambiguous language it used and the fact that it seemed to offer something to everyone. It also solidified hopes raised by Winterton and then seemingly dashed by the response of the government. Finally, it chimed with wider government philosophies about choice within the NHS as well as offering a low-cost alternative to hospital-based consultant-driven care; another central tenet of the Conservative government's belief. The Report was not just significant for the way it spoke to government, however. It held out the promise of a better world for both service users and service providers. In journal reports and newspaper articles there is a sense from both of these groups that after years of obstetric hegemony their voices were at last being heard and their viewpoints recognised. AIMS and the NCT – involved not only in giving evidence, but in shaping the Report – evinced a belief that when implemented, its recommendations would bring about wholesale change in the maternity services (NCT 1996). For midwives the lure was, if anything, even stronger.

The Report held out the promise of midwives using what they perceived to be their full range of professional skills, rather than functioning simply as what were described by some as: obstetric handmaidens. Articles were written, conferences convened and books and manuals developed, all with the aim of putting the midwife back, as it was seen, at the centre of maternity. Walton and Hamilton, two midwifery educators, wrote a whole book on the subject in 1995. They summed up the promise of the Report:

> Throughout the 1970s and 1980s it appeared that technology was rapidly taking over the care of the childbearing woman. Midwives were becoming little more than technicians in the process and the woman herself was becoming unnoticed in the pursuit of the visibility and importance of the fetus ... As two midwives living through this era, and its inherent frustrations, the possibility of reports such as 'Winterton' and 'Changing Childbirth' seemed beyond the realms of probability ...
>
> 'Changing Childbirth' represents a unique opportunity for all professionals involved in the delivery of maternity care to work together to enable women to have choice, control, continuity, and ultimately, satisfaction with their experiences ...
>
> (Walton and Hamilton 1995: vi)

They argued, moreover, that 'this opportunity will not present itself again'.

Mavis Kirkham, an active researcher and writer at the time, as well as a midwife, recalled this sense of a new dawn offered by *Changing Childbirth*, not just in terms of what it seemed to offer in the way of practical change, but equally significantly, in the way in which it opened up debate:

> There was a really strong feeling that there was hope. It strengthened a lot of people; it kept a lot of people in midwifery who would otherwise have left in despair at that point. And there was this lovely short period where there were lots of continuity of care pilot projects which were funded, and they worked. And I was involved in one but it was axed before we finished the evaluation. And it was a privilege to be involved in it, but it was a very interesting era because you were getting very open debate with the people who were saying, this won't work managerially and women can't have choice and what's the point in training to be a midwife if we don't know best. So all this was happening and it was a

very exciting time to be writing and doing research because you'd got articles in the midwifery press saying this won't work signed by named managers, senior managers in midwifery, which you wouldn't get nowadays because everybody's so skilled in the double speak now, nobody would write like that.

(Mavis Kirkham interview)

The window, as Kirkham saw it, was brief as it became clear that, however impassioned and powerful the debate, choice and control did remain primarily with doctors, managers and risk assessors even though Page (1992) suggested that the Report had 'deep human wisdom'.

Changing Childbirth had an emotional legacy both for women's groups and for midwives. It also had practical elements, including the development of *Informed Choice* leaflets for women, of templates for birth plans and a raft of publications and new editions, describing to women how they could ensure that they had 'choice' and 'control' in pregnancy and birth (Anderson 1995; Wesson 1995; Thomas 1996, 1998). For midwives it resulted in debate about what constituted the role, and about wider skills development. Much of this was driven not just by *Changing Childbirth* and by philosophical beliefs, but by practical necessity, including the European Union Working Time Directive which impacted on the hours that doctors could work. Some areas and some midwives embraced concepts of team midwifery and the promised impact of less fragmented care; although there was a variety of different language used to describe these concepts (Flint 1993; Stock and Wraight 1993; Page 1995; Lee 1997; Perkins and Unell 1997; Walker 1996, 1999). There were, however, warning notes particularly around the desire and desirability of midwives to work in that way and concerns about physical and emotional burn-out (Sandall 1997). Not all midwives welcomed the potential loss of structure to their working lives; there was a sense that they too wanted control and that it might conflict with that of women (Brain 1991). One correspondent to the *Midwives Chronicle* commented that 'Not all [midwives] want, or are able, to return to the days of five nights out of seven on call with no personal life'. The General Secretary of the RCM commented soon after the publication of the Winterton Report that the work of midwives had been compartmentalised into 'neatly packaged shift systems' and that change would mean midwives taking responsibility for their decisions and their actions (Ashton 1992). Despite reports and schemes for different ways of working, which appeared both before and after *Changing Childbirth*, shift work continued to be the dominant pattern of midwifery working (Gifford 1996). There was debate as to whether vested interests prevented novel schemes of care being implemented, but even more that changes were piecemeal and poorly evaluated (Jowitt 1998).

The placing in the mainstream of debate of such words as 'choice' and 'control' belied the fact that they meant different things to different people.

Although the concepts were taken up by 'radical' midwives and the great and good of the RCM alike (not necessarily different people), they were also part of a wider market-driven view of society. There was little contemporary critique even from radical midwives of the relevance of capitalist buzz words to pregnancy and birth. Some debated anxiously the fact that the logical conclusion of maternal choice was that women could make the decision to have a Caesarean section, for example, with no references to the possible risks (McAleese 2000).

Finally, it could be argued that although *Changing Childbirth* gave impetus to debates in midwifery and excitement to many consumer groups, it was essentially the flowering of a middle-class view of childbirth, codified by AIMS and the NCT. Working-class women did not necessarily use the same language about birth, or hold the same beliefs (McIntosh 1989; Perkins 1991). Work by McIntosh in Glasgow suggested that for many women, birth was something to be dealt with on the way to motherhood with very little expression of a belief in a 'natural' experience. For the majority of women in his survey, the availability of pain relief was the primary concern. The idea that women had a homogeneous view of birth was gradually being challenged (Nelson 1983) but this did not feed into *Changing Childbirth* or the debate surrounding it.

Midwives were no more homogeneous than women. There was a sense among some that *Changing Childbirth* devalued the midwife by putting so much emphasis on the power of the consumer. There was also a feeling that everything that had gone before was seen to be wrong, which left some midwives feeling that they had lost more than they had gained. One community midwife explained this sense not of hope but of loss engendered by *Changing Childbirth*:

> However, it seemed that the community way of practising was old fashioned and a new way had to be found without ever looking back. We sat on a working party to find a new way forward. We drew up a plan to incorporate the whole of the hospital and combine it with the community. The plan was centred on the mother and would give all midwives the chance to work together with midwives on the community. A new manager arrived and our plan was torn up without ever being implemented. At great expense, we then tried out many of the new team approaches which had been introduced around the country. One by one they were discarded but it was too late, very large teams were now the way forward, whether they worked or not, they are composed of newly qualified midwives and slightly more experienced midwives and one G grade per team. On calls all the time and according to my colleagues and young mums who I am still in contact with, very little continuity as before. The midwives seem to be forever coming and going and are a little disillusioned with things.
>
> (Eustance 2000)

Another commented on what she saw as the emptiness of the promises made to both mothers and midwives:

> Changing Childbirth was heralded as the best thing that could ever happen to childbirth. It seemed to mean that mothers would be spoilt for choice of care, carer and place to deliver her baby. In short, this was the revolution that mothers and midwives were waiting for.
>
> Sadly, I see and hear that most women have little real choice in the decision making process. The choice is which day would you like to be induced, and not a discussion about the pros and cons of induction and the woman making an informed decision. Women automatically become part of routine care the minute they are booked.
>
> Another area of confusion is in the dishonest promotion of informed choice. What if women choose not to have continuous fetal monitoring in labour? Many protocols state that a routine admission trace must be performed and if the woman declines it must be recorded in her notes. I feel so passionately that childbirth should be returned to mothers but this cannot take place while all the fears and myths continue to be dangled in front of them from the very start of pregnancy. This attitude tells her who is really running the show. Women truly need to be empowered with knowledge so they can learn to trust their bodies and be enabled to allow their natural instincts to play their part.
>
> Has anything changed in childbirth for the midwife? I don't want to be too negative; there have been some changes. But the introduction of team midwifery brought with it downgrading of midwives' posts and relocation of the working base. It brought changes of shift patterns and a flexibility that has created sleepless nights and variable working hours that leave midwives with little family or social life. There is a palpable atmosphere of fear of losing one's job if one doesn't adapt and change to fit in. The style of management seems to have developed for the worse, management don't seem to care as once they did; they have become focused on money.
>
> (Watts 1997)

It could therefore be argued that the reception of *Changing Childbirth* and other reports gave only an illusion of change and improvement. The implementation of midwifery-led units, with their highly structured criteria of 'risk', or the provision on the NHS of birthing balls, pools or complementary therapies suggested that women's demands and choices were central to service provision. At the same time, however, beliefs about risk were tightly drawn, and intervention rates, particularly as regards Caesareans, continued to climb (the Caesarean rate was 4 per cent in 1970, rising to 9 per cent in 1980 and 21.5 per cent by 2000: Birth Choice UK 2012).

In summary, the Winterton and *Changing Childbirth* Reports have been discussed in detail because they did represent a change in the terms of the debate around maternity service provision, and rippled out more widely than just managers or professionals. The language and tenets of *Changing Child-birth* have echoed down through contemporary reports and beliefs about practice, with ideas of 'choice' and 'control' seen as unarguably positive. The concept was not at the time as revolutionary as it has been seen, but in many ways merely codified debate and change which was already occurring. Its power lay in its use of language and the fact that it seemed to offer something to everyone involved in maternity. Its legacy has, however, been mixed with hope which seemingly turned quickly to disillusion as many of the schemes created in its wake floundered for want of sustained backing both financial and psychological. Its recommendations did not chime with all midwives or all women. Concepts of choice and control and even continuity were arguably fundamentally flawed in the context of maternity (Stapleton 1997) where there were always things that could not be controlled, whatever the systems in place. Women also had to have the freedom and right to choose things which professionals would not have them choose; whether it was a home birth after a previous Caesarean section, or a Caesarean section with no apparent obstetric need. Giving women choice meant giving them the right to make the 'wrong' choices; something that professionals, both doctors and midwives, found very hard to swallow. As Symon (2006) argued, it was during this period that the concept of 'risk' seriously came to be embedded in maternity care. *Changing Childbirth* stepped back from the debates around safety in maternity, particularly as regards the home versus hospital debate, and did not use the word 'risk' at all. Nevertheless, it seems to have been something of a lifeline for professionals in the face of the deluge of official support for women's choice. As commentators have argued, 'risk' is a concept as slippery and value laden as 'choice' and as easily open to interpretation (Walsh 2003).

Research and education

One of the tenets on which *Changing Childbirth* was based was that of the provision of research evidence on which to base everything from national policy to individual decisions, a development which was surprisingly new. Maternity services in England developed across the twentieth century in response to a variety of internal and external pressures. These included the needs and expectations of service users and of wider society as well as developments in technology or changes in workforce, training or management. In the last 20 years of the period a new agent for change appeared, however, as research by midwives and others moved from a minority activity to the mainstream of education and debate. This section will explore the background to this development, how research came to be embedded in the midwifery professional project in particular, and the impact of this on practice and on the wider profession.

Research is characterised as systematic enquiry into an identified problem or question which follows a logical and replicable process in order to reach its conclusions. In some guises research has always been utilised within the maternity services whether clinically, epidemically or socially focused. Thus, explorations into puerperal fever, the perinatal mortality surveys, or the investigations by Llewelyn Davies into the maternity experiences of working women, are all examples of different types of evidence brought to bear on maternity care.

There was a broad change in ideas around research which developed in the early 1970s, when it came to be seen as a possible panacea for perceived problems in maternity care for a variety of reasons. The first was systemic; midwives and nurses were encouraged not just passively to absorb ideas about care but to become actively involved in research. The impetus for this came from the Briggs Report (1972) which was primarily concerned with the operational aspects of the move towards an integrated health service leading up to the 1974 reorganisation of the NHS. Within this, the Report made a significant statement about the centrality of research to nursing and midwifery practice:

> We have been given ample evidence that in nursing and midwifery education insufficient attention is paid to research as a continuing activity. Nor is there enough emphasis on research as a prelude to innovation. Nursing should become a research-based profession ... a sense of the need for research should become part of the mental equipment of every practising nurse or midwife.
>
> (Briggs Report 1972: 108)

The Report drew attention to nursing research already in progress. This revolved around issues of management, communication and education, with no evidence presented of either clinical or midwifery research.

The call by the Briggs Report chimed with another by epidemiologist Archie Cochrane whose work *Effectiveness and Efficiency: Random Reflections on the Health Service* (1972) pilloried the maternity services in particular for the enthusiastic and wholesale take up of technologies and techniques which had no real research back-up. Cochrane has been credited with being one of the founders of 'evidence-based care' although the phrase itself did not appear in the literature until the early 1990s (Guyatt 1992). Research into aspects of midwifery practice developed during the 1970s with influential work being done around the issue of induction of labour in particular. Research papers appeared in medical journals which discussed and critiqued obstetric practice, but none of this was done by midwives. Beyond the work of doctors, important and eye-catching research into maternity was conducted by those outside the profession, including anthropologists (Kitzinger), sociologists (Oakley, Cartwright), statisticians (Tew and Macfarlane) and, as noted, lay members of consumer groups such as Robinson. Iain Chalmers, Director of the NPEU, drew attention to the contribution of these researchers to maternity, and the wider impact that this debate had on the development of new ideas around social medicine and public health (Berridge et al. 2006). The research that was done set the tone of debate around practice and service configuration which fed into reports such as *Changing Childbirth*.

It was a variety of factors which finally prompted some midwives to develop their research awareness, and in particular, although the focus on external drivers for research, including service improvement suggested by Briggs and Cochrane, did not appear to impact on midwives, internal drivers did. Allison (interview) suggested that the involvement of midwives such as herself in research came as a direct result of changes in the structure of the service and the perceived de-skilling of midwives. She argued that, on a personal level, she needed to understand why midwifery was floundering as a profession, and research seemed to be the best tool with which to explore this.

By the early 1980s there was a small community of midwives who were beginning to describe themselves as researchers, and there is a sense that they were working to encourage each other and build up a belief in the efficacy of research (Kirkham 1981). The substance of the research that was developed was very much influenced by the agenda set by researchers external to midwifery, and by the internal beliefs about professional status. It was largely characterised by a women-centred and feminist stance. Clark (2000) argued that the growth of midwifery research has resulted in ' … the development of a sound knowledge base for maternity care' and furthermore that 'without research evidence it is difficult to differentiate between unsubstantiated prejudice and reliable knowledge.' This is to offer very much a Whig interpretation of research, implying that care before its advent was likely to be of dubious quality and efficacy. Although feminist researchers in particular (Oakley 1981b) had a tradition of acknowledging the partiality and prejudices inherent in research, acceptance of research by the midwifery community very much followed Clark's interpretation, with research evidence being viewed as a positive platform for care, and anything else as based on 'tradition', which was seen, not least by the *Changing Childbirth* Report, as an inadequate basis for care. In the introduction to their first volume *Midwives, Research and Childbirth* (1989), editors Sarah Robinson and Ann Thomson commented that: 'During the 1970s, the view steadily gained ground that midwifery practice and education should be based on research findings rather than on custom and tradition or the dictates of other professional groups' (Robinson and Thomson 1989: 2). Unpicking this statement, it is clear that research in midwifery had its initial impetus from ideas around practice, but even more powerfully from beliefs about professional status. Research would give midwives the professional standing which some felt would come from engaging with obstetricians on their own terms. In order to do this opposition had to be created, between research which was seen as good and 'traditional' which was seen as bad. Emerging midwifery researchers devalued the work and lives of those who had come before them by implying that only through research could midwives be effective. In doing so they allied themselves to a reductionist view which suggested, ultimately, that only that which could be counted mattered. Although midwife researchers argued that they changed the terms of the debate, they could be seen as ceding final power to medicine, by discrediting midwifery forms of knowledge. Brenda, who worked in the 1960s and 1970s, described knowledge as being passed down from 'the old spinster midwives' and described practices such as putting cabbage leaves on engorged breasts, which she felt worked, but which were unproven by science. She linked the rise in research-based midwifery to the rise in potential litigation:

> Yes, I mean with the cord stump, some midwives used to have ... it was like a blue stone and they used to put this blue stone, rub this blue stone on the stump, and it used to just miraculously heal. I never used it because I was never taught with it, but I know it worked, because there was one midwife who always used it and they always cleared up. So I think there is a place for some things to be brought back, but as I say, litigation will never allow it.

(Brenda interview)

Several early pieces of midwifery research were focused not only on clinical questions but on the development and hegemony of midwifery itself. This could be seen as an attempt to push a particular professional agenda at a time of flux for the maternity services. Midwives such as Allison were drawn to research as a way of saving their profession from what they saw as potential extinction. Research projects included those which considered the role and training of students (Mander 1983; Robinson 1991), and the contribution of midwives to care; in particular the thorny question of the extent to which they were being de-skilled (Robinson 1980; Bradley et al. 1981; Henderson 1984; Garcia et al. 1985). The influence of non-midwifery research was clear in the tenor of research by midwives which explored the relationship between women and care givers (Methven 1982; Kirkham 1989) and women's attitudes to care offered (Kirchmeier 1984).

Midwifery research fed into the belief in evidence-based practice which continued to develop in the 1980s. Cochrane's strictures on the maternity service and its use of evidence were instrumental in, and celebrated by, the development of the Cochrane Review. This began life as a systematic trawling of research literature on pregnancy and birth from the 1950s onwards, and eventually resulted in a two-volume review and an electronic database. This database is now considered to be a model of the use of research evidence, and its conclusions inform policies and guidelines across the country. The belief in the need for all practitioners to be research aware was shown in the publication of a smaller volume (Chalmers et al. 1989) which was to be used by 'all who are involved in the care of childbearing women' (Enkin et al. 1995: vii). The team involved included a midwife as well as obstetricians, and drew up recommendations for practice based on whether or not a treatment or intervention was deemed to be beneficial, harmful or neutral. The concept of 'doing the sick no harm' on which the layout drew was an ancient one, first described by Hippocrates (Porter 1997). Although there was some discussion of psycho-social interventions in pregnancy and birth, the majority of the recommendations were based on clinical indicators, more easily measured by an experimental methodology such as a randomised controlled trial. Research with a social science bent, such as that based on ethnography or phenomenology, was harder to fit into the objective criteria which quantitative research seemed to offer. There have been critiques of the role of research in maternity care, and in particular the over-reliance on experimental methodologies rather than those which put experience and belief at the centre of the study. Many early midwife researchers came from a social science background (for example Kirkham) and gravitated towards qualitative research. Once again, however, they found themselves marginalised by a system which valued quantitative research above all else, and at times seemed to relegate qualitative approaches to the status of the 'tradition' that midwife researchers claimed to be trying to get away from.

In 1985 midwives associated with ARM set up the Midwives Information and Resource Service (MIDIRS) with the same remit as that suggested by Robinson and Thomson: that midwives needed research knowledge in order to develop as a profession and to challenge obstetric practice (Kargar 1996; Anderson 2006). The intention of the service was to produce a journal summarising significant research which had appeared in a range of other journals, and to produce information packs detailing references on a variety of topics for use by midwifery students and researchers. The development of research databases, such as that started on a small scale by MIDIRS, relied on a constant output of relevant research. From the late 1970s a large proportion both of studies and of expertise came from the National Perinatal Epidemiology Unit (NPEU) which was established in 1978 under the auspices of the University of Oxford. The Unit was led by Iain Chalmers, and contained many of the same personnel as those involved in the Cochrane database. Clark (2000) argued that these research initiatives not only impacted on care, but that the support they gave to researchers allowed expertise to ripple out. Certainly internationally recognised midwifery researchers such as Mary Renfrew, who began her work with Cochrane and the NPEU, went on to establish significant research groups in their own right. Research which impacted significantly on the care given to women, such as that by Sleep et al. (1983, 1984, 1991) on routine and elective episiotomies, was supported by the NPEU. Clark (2000) delineated some of the main pieces of midwifery-based research conducted in the early 1980s, some of which, including that of Sleep, attained almost iconic status in the midwifery canon.

However important the research project, it was meaningless without dissemination. Engaging the 'ordinary' midwife with research was one of the challenges and was carried out through a variety of mediums with varying degrees of success. Individual projects were traditionally presented orally to interested colleagues, then formally through written papers, and finally through inclusion on databases. Dissemination more broadly followed this trajectory. Midwifery research conferences began in the late 1970s, with the first one being developed by Robinson and Thomson in 1978. Papers given were published first in conference proceedings and by the late 1980s as more formal edited volumes (Robinson and Thomson 1989). This was the forum through which many of the first cohort of midwifery researchers found their voice, and were increasingly well attended with 220 delegates attending the conference of 1981 (Grant 1981). They were not the only ones engaging with research however. ARM, who developed MIDIRS, showcased research findings from the time of its first conference in 1981; including the seminal work of Mona Romney on perineal shaving, which took women's voices as its rationale for undertaking the study:

> At a time of increased consumer participation in medical and nursing matters, a variety of obstetric procedures have been criticised by the lay public. It is clear that shaving is unpopular with the patient, and it is in the interest of Medical and Nursing staff concerned with obstetrics, either to justify the procedure on medical grounds, or comply with the patient's wishes and abandon it.
>
> (Romney 1981)

The lingering influence of earlier attitudes can clearly be seen in the language used, particularly around the oppositional nature of the relationship between 'patients' and 'medicine'.

In 1985 a new journal for midwives was founded. Called simply *Midwifery* its aim was to be 'an international forum where [midwives] could exchange ideas, share and extend knowledge and participate in debate' although it did hope for 'original research' to be submitted through articles and letters, almost in the style of a medical journal. Midwives had hitherto relied on 'the Chron' the *Midwives Chronicle* which was produced monthly by the RCM and posted out to all its members. It too was slowly developing research awareness, and gave a platform to early midwifery researchers such as Robinson (1981; Bradley et al. 1981). Further publications followed: *Modern Midwife* (later *The Practising Midwife*) in 1991 followed by the *British Journal of Midwifery* in 1993. These journals relied on a growing number of midwives willing and able to write for publication, and on a population of midwives interested in reading their work. One of the ideas they sought to promulgate was around the survival and furtherance of the profession. Kirkman (1994) argued that midwives needed to develop their own body of research, and therefore of knowledge, to conform to classic ideas of what constituted a profession. This suggests that far from growing in self-confidence as a separate profession, midwives took on board the medical discourse around what constituted authoritative knowledge. The belief in research was supported by the CMB and the RCM but it did prove decisive for midwives in many ways. Quite apart from anything else, it could be used, deliberately or otherwise, as a stick with which to beat midwives. Beverley Beech (1992), the Chair of AIMS, argued that despite their research, midwives were continuing to undertake procedures which were unethical because they were unproven. Taken to its logical conclusion; this suggested that everything a midwife did should first be subjected to research, a belief that potentially undermined the professional status of the midwife. An editorial in *Midwifery* argued that research needed to be conducted as 'systematic scientific enquiry' (June 1985) implying a lack of self-belief in other forms of professional knowledge and understanding. Interestingly, however, midwifery researchers could not take a belief in their work by other midwives as read; one study demonstrated that midwives valued work which they believed to have been done by obstetricians more highly than that believed to have been done by midwives (Hicks 1992).

Many of the early research projects conducted by midwives were based around issues from practice or perceptions of service. The move of midwives into higher and research degrees took place very slowly. The first PhD in midwifery was awarded in 1982, and by 1998 only a handful of midwives had research degrees (Clark 2000). Below this, however, midwifery education was expanding with the development of both degree and Master level programmes, initially in conjunction with universities and eventually, as nursing and midwifery became absorbed into higher education, wholly through them. Midwifery education ceased to be conducted by a multiplicity of training colleges linked to hospitals and moved into university premises, with educational quality now the responsible of the English National Board. For some midwives the development meant not only that they could see themselves alongside doctors in particular in terms of professional status, but also that they would be held in 'greater public esteem' (Ward and Adams 1979) although others argued that midwives with degrees could find themselves marginalised within the profession.

In conjunction with these developments, the profession was once again looking at the provision of midwifery training vis-à-vis that of nursing. In 1988 a Report by Radford and Thompson explored the possibility of developing 'direct entry' training for midwives. Midwives had never been required to first undertake nurse training, despite it being recommended reluctantly by the Stocks Report of 1949 and more enthusiastically by the Briggs Report of 1972. However, the vast majority of midwives were also nurses, and by the mid-1980s it was very hard for a student to achieve the status of midwife without first being a nurse. Just as the Stocks Report had noted in 1949, this led to problems of retention, as a relatively small proportion of nurse qualified midwives stayed in the role. For most it was a stepping stone to management or health visiting. However, midwifery had fought the proposals of the Briggs Report for an 18-month common foundation programme in nursing, followed by a further 18 months for those wanting to specialise in midwifery, and had managed to have midwifery removed from the planning for Project 2000 which aimed to develop a common foundation curriculum across nursing specialities (Radford and Thompson 1988: 45). The resurgence of midwifery interest in Direct Entry training was, like the development of midwifery research, another attempt to re-focus the concept of a midwifery 'profession' distinct from nursing and medicine. It was argued that non-nurse midwives would be more focused on normality, as opposed to concepts of pathology inculcated by nurse training, and would stand up more determinedly for the profession of midwifery. Support for Direct Entry training meant that by the end of the period, for the first time since midwifery training had been developed, a substantial proportion of midwives had no nursing background. This caused debate about the effectiveness and competence of non-nurse midwives (Dike 2005). One midwife who trained in the mid-1990s recalled that:

> I was a direct entry midwife and was greeted by midwives in my place of training with anything from 'you're not getting the best training' to 'well, paper qualifications mean nothing'. Experience is a wonderful quality I agree but I didn't make the rules, I didn't decide how midwives were to be trained and all I asked was for my mentors to pass on their wealth of experience in the hope I would make a half decent midwife.
> I was, and still am, to a point, made to feel like a second class midwife.
>
> (Gail, Midwifery Matters Forum)

The UKCC, the national regulatory body which succeeded the CMB and regional nursing boards in 1979, had codified a level of takeover of midwifery by nursing, since midwifery was no longer governed or regulated separately. In 2002, in a different climate, the UKCC was itself abolished in favour of the NMC, which intended to give a stronger voice to midwifery. However, to the disappointment of campaigners, midwifery was still just one part of a broader nursing council, however persistent its belief in its own profession project.

Obstetrics triumphant?

Despite all the debates about consumer choice and midwifery hegemony, despite a resurgence of interest in natural and active birth, the clearest sign that technology was winning the battle for childbirth was the rising Caesarean section rate, and the proliferation in indications for its use. In the 10th edition of *Mayes' Midwifery* textbook, published in 1984, it was commented that although a Caesarean delivery carried a higher death rate than a normal delivery it was safer for mother and baby than a 'very difficult vaginal delivery'; there was no evidence suggested for this statement (Sweet 1984: 383). Indications for performing a section included 'prolonged labour', 'maternal or fetal distress before second stage' and malpresentations, including breech, alongside issues such as placenta praevia or pelvic disproportion. By the publication of the 11th edition of Sweet's book in 1988 the indications included previous Caesarean; a situation which would inevitably cause the rate to rise as every first Caesarean would potentially lead to others. At this point, however, the rate of section deliveries, although climbing, was not a cause for official or even midwifery alarm. Caesareans had accounted for 2.2 per cent of deliveries in 1953, and were still less than 5 per cent in 1973, reflecting obstetric concern about the risks of the procedures and obstetric confidence in other ways of handling complex situations. Despite the move of birth from home to hospital, and the explosion of belief in the induction of labour, the Caesarean section rate did not reach double figures until 1982 (Macfarlane et al. 2000). Twelve years later the rate had reached 15.5 per cent nationally, and a breakdown of the figures demonstrates changing beliefs about risk and safety; in 1979 4.5 per cent of Caesareans had been 'elective' and 3.7 per cent 'emergency'. 'Elective' was traditionally taken to mean that the decision for Caesarean delivery was taken prior to labour, in contrast to an 'emergency' where the decision was taken in response to events in labour (when the decision to operation interval could be as little as ten minutes). By 1994/95, however, the relative positions of elective and emergency indications were reversed, which suggests both an increase in the perceived indications for emergency bailout and the growth in the use of technology to guide decision making. The development of CTG monitoring, to pictorially indicate foetal heart rate patterns, together with foetal blood sampling to give an idea of potential hypoxia, certainly contributed to the rush to theatre. However contentious accuracy or interpretation was, once something 'abnormal' was detected it had to be acted on, if only to stave off fears of litigation. Despite the publication around this time of *Changing Childbirth* with its re-emphasis on normality, Caesarean births continued to increase at a rate of 1 per cent a year, reaching 22 per cent nationally in 2001/2, and varying from 24.2 per cent in London to 19.3 per cent in the North-East of England (Paranjothy and Thomas 2001).

In response to this rise a national audit was carried out under the joint auspices of the RCOG, the RCM, the Royal College of Anaesthetists and the NCT: the *Sentinel Audit* (Paranjothy and Thomas 2001). As befitting the post-*Changing Childbirth* era, the audit canvassed the views of women as well as those of professionals. The report noted that women who responded to its questionnaire were more likely to be white, older and in their first pregnancy than the general maternity population. It was noted that one of the beliefs about the rising Caesarean rate was that it in itself mushroomed after *Changing Childbirth* and the foregrounding of women's right to choose. For some women, it seemed, this meant exercising their right to choose a Caesarean section. Research found this problematic to assess, because concepts of 'maternal request' varied widely, depending on whether medical, psychological and emotional factors were included. Despite the fears of newspaper headline writers, the *Sentinel Audit* did not support the contention that women were demanding Caesareans either for convenience or because they were 'too posh to push' (Paranjothy and Thomas 2001). However, it did throw up some contradictions. The evidence suggested that the majority of women surveyed wanted birth to be as natural as possible, but at the same time wanted it to be as pain free as possible. They also wanted to be in control of the process whilst contending that the safety of the baby was of paramount importance. Beyond that, the belief that women had a right to a Caesarean whatever the circumstances was stronger than a concomitant belief in the right to a vaginal birth. Given the wide variation in rates between regions, hospitals and individual consultants, debates and decisions were clearly taking place on a very personal basis, and are likely to have been informed by a multiplicity of factors. Similar, if broader, findings had come from a study of women's expectations around birth, conducted in 1987, but published in the wake of *Changing Childbirth* (Green et al. 1998). None of the authors were midwives or doctors, but they echoed the confusion of these groups in delineating the contradictions inherent in the beliefs that women held about birth in particular. The study argued that, contrary to received wisdom, highly educated women were not necessarily anti-technology, intervention or pain relief, and women from lower social groups were at least as likely to want natural births. The authors pointed, however, to the contradictions inherent in the concepts of 'choice' and 'control'; they meant different things to different people, with 'choice' in particular being constrained by what individuals thought might be possible.

It was not only consumers who struggled with the semantics of choice and control; the *Sentinel Audit* demonstrated the extent to which doctors felt they lacked control over rising rates of Caesarean births. Over half of those surveyed felt that current levels were too high, but despite their status as consultants felt powerless to tackle it in a meaningful way. This suggests that broader beliefs were at play, not just about the rights of women to demand the birth experience of their choice *pace Changing Childbirth*, but also around the vexed question of litigation and risk. Various explanations have been suggested for the growth in what is described as defensive practice by clinicians and the associated growth in claims by families. The use of Legal Aid for fighting cases on behalf of infants was sanctioned after 1990, and this could be seen as having an impact on claims, which tended to be based on intra-partum issues, and therefore on the development of practices which professionals felt that they could defend, including Caesarean sections. Paradoxically, the situation may have been exacerbated by consumer campaigners, particularly Robinson and Beech of AIMS who set up the Maternity Defence Fund which actively sought out women who had had what could be argued as unnecessary procedures, with the intention of suing the obstetrician. The Fund was intended to be one way to strip obstetricians of their power and remind them of their responsibilities, and also to bring to the fore an understanding by professionals of the significance of informed consent for procedures (Finch 1982; Robinson 1982). Beech did admit, however, that one of the unintended consequences may be an increase in the practice of defensive obstetrics (*The Times* 11.09.1985). Cameron and Ellwood (2006) argued that the conflation of Caesarean birth with lower risk, and therefore its growth, were related particularly to trials which compared vaginal delivery and found the former wanting. The most famous, and contested, example of this was the Hannah breech trial (2000) which suggested that Caesarean section was safer than vaginal birth for babies presenting by the breech, and which therefore gave the impression that a Caesarean could be a low-risk option in some cases. The arguments around the relative safety of vaginal and Caesarean birth mirrored those around home and hospital birth 30 years previously, with the differing views equally irreconcilable.

Conclusion

The final years of the twentieth century saw a wholesale change in the language used about maternity by all of those who had some involvement whether as consumers, policy makers or professionals. The language of choice, control and consent was increasingly used both before, but particularly after, *Changing Childbirth*. This report argued that the medicalisation of birth had gone too far, and that for the majority of women a highly technological birth was neither necessary nor desirable. Midwives used the impetus of *Changing Childbirth* to recast their professional identity, and were largely successful in being characterised as the 'lead professional' in normal pregnancy and birth. This chapter has touched on only a fraction of the debates which were occurring in the maternity services during this period; it has not considered the impact of increase in delayed motherhood or the impact of assisted conception and fertility treatment on beliefs and expectations around maternity, for example. It has highlighted, nevertheless, that for all the rhetoric about natural birth and choice, it was the language of science, technology and risk which was winning by the turn of the new millennium. Whatever the significance of groups such as the Active Birth Movement or the beliefs evinced by *Changing Childbirth*, it was the Caesarean section rate, inexorably rising, which seemed to give the lie to consumer and midwifery power.

Conclusion

This book has taken a broad sweep through the history of maternity care in twentieth-century England in order to delineate some of the main features of the landscape. Pregnancy and birth are uniquely public and private at the same time; significant to individuals and families, and also to society in its widest sense. They also exist at the interface between medical and social discourse, and it is this which has caused some of the most significant debates around maternity across the century. At different points society and medicine have taken on varying levels of prescription around pregnancy and birth, whether related to concerns about infant or maternal health, the rising or falling birth rate, or the interface between mother and foetus and whose health and rights should be paramount. These complexities impacted on both policy decisions and day-to-day beliefs about pregnancy and birth.

The story of maternity has often been elided with that of midwifery, and told as a struggle for power and influence between (female) midwives and (male) doctors. This has been evinced in tales of professional rivalry, of technological development, and in the battle over the place of birth. Within these histories women, as mothers, have tended to be invisible, subsumed into a wider battle for control over childbirth.

However, this work has used a variety of evidence, both secondary and primary, to demonstrate that the story of maternity in twentieth-century England is far more nuanced than it first appears. To begin with, it is clear that women of all classes had power and agency throughout the period. Women continued to patronise untrained midwives for many years after the 1902 Act because untrained midwives would cook and clean and help to sustain the household. They campaigned for the right to use analgesia for labour, and for the right to give birth in hospital. Then, in the second half of the twentieth century women argued for more, and less, intervention. They demanded active birth and epidurals, natural births and continuity of care. Some of this was done through specific organisations such as Women's Co-operative Guild or the NCT, but some of it was achieved through individual conversations and actions. The consumer movement in maternity really developed from the 1960s onwards, and had a significant impact on the language and beliefs developed around birth by policy makers and professionals. But women had

had a voice throughout the twentieth century, and their demands for services such as hospital birth had shaped policy and provision across the decades. It was, however, a voice which was sometimes contradictory, and for health professionals and policy makers there could sometimes be heard the plaintive cry of 'what do women actually want?'

The traditional argument that maternity services developed in the way that they did as a result of professional rivalries between doctors and midwives underplays the extent to which the groups had common ground, and furthermore the extent to which their roles developed in the twentieth century. Individual relationships between doctors and midwives were not necessarily oppositional; there is a wealth of evidence detailing their ability to work together, regardless of the broader rhetoric about rivalries. Across the period doctors respected the work that midwives did, and relations between GPs and midwives in particular could be mutually supportive. This belies the fact, however, that it was not midwives who lost the battle to be regarded as professionals in the field of birth; it was GPs. It was the GP who was vilified across the period, being accused of responsibility for infection and maternal death in the inter-war years, and for high rates of perinatal mortality in the post-war years. They were castigated as generalists who could not be trusted to put on a pair of forceps or send for help. The battle, therefore, was between the specialists – in the guise of midwives and obstetricians – and GPs. The GPs clearly lost. At the beginning of the twentieth century GPs retained significant involvement in childbirth, and they continued to campaign for it to be seen as a domestic, family affair, ideally suited to the ministrations of a family doctor. However, they did this at a time first of official concern over maternal death rates, for which they were blamed, and which therefore gave them little leverage. In the post-war period, once antibiotics and blood transfusions had seemingly defeated the scourge of maternal deaths, GPs tried once again. This time, however, it was women who wanted to deliver in hospital, and midwives, who had their own profession to defend, who did not make common cause with GPs. By the 1980s the battle was largely lost and while GPs continued to play a diminished role in antenatal care provision, they were very unlikely to be part of intra-partum or even postnatal care.

GPs were squeezed out of care by midwives and by obstetricians who staked their own claims across the period for rights over the territory of childbirth and carved it up between them. By the time of the publication of *Changing Childbirth* in 1993, maternity had been divided into 'normal' and 'abnormal', 'high risk' and 'low risk'. Midwives controlled anything considered to be normal and obstetricians took the rest. In doing so both groups had reinvented themselves; they were not monolithic entities across the period. In 1902 a midwife was likely to be middle aged, married or widowed, unlikely to be trained and likely to ply her trade primarily among working-class clients. She was independently employed, relying on the fees scraped together by her clients. Even 20 years later many of the same features remained, with the majority of midwives still untrained and poorly remunerated, with only a handful of cases to sustain them. Despite the work of successive governments midwives did not play a significant part in the antenatal care or ideas about public health. In the second half of the century, however, they reinvented themselves through training, salaried employment and a growing confidence in their qualities, particularly in relation to the much maligned GP. Overworked and underpaid they may have been, but midwives repositioned themselves as professionals focused on the normal. This was achieved not just through their own efforts, but through those of government, both national and local, and obstetricians, to sanitise their work. Midwives in the post-war period prided themselves on being with women, but their perceived status as professionals was at least as important to them. Relations between midwives and women became increasingly strained across the period as training and education, and perceptions about their status took midwives further away from many women. The issue became more acute with the development of a consumer voice by women from the 1970s, with both midwives and women denigrating each other's position, and struggling to find common cause.

Midwives were not the only ones who rewrote their job descriptions and developed their roles across the period. Obstetricians had developed from those generalist GPs they so despised, although until the last decades of the century, their work centred on heroics in the second stage of a labour rather than any finesse over care. From the 1960s onwards obstetricians repositioned themselves not just as heroes who wrested a live mother and baby from a hopeless situation, but as professionals who had hegemony over the whole span of pregnancy and birth. They were assisted in this by the development of technology which gave them control over the situation: scans to date pregnancy and chart the growth of the hitherto hidden baby, drugs and instruments to induce and then limit labour, and if all else failed, an increasing confidence with the previously nerve-wracking operation of a Caesarean section. Although it could be seen as professional grandstanding, issues such as maternal death cast a long shadow over the beliefs and practices of obstetricians, however.

Mothers, midwives and doctors were all individuals with different beliefs and ideas which sometimes chimed with and were sometimes at odds with the prevailing mood. Ideas of choice and control, which were foregrounded in the last decade of the twentieth century by *Changing Childbirth*, actually applied across the period and to all groups, whether in relation to birth itself, or in the case of doctors and midwives, to issues around their working lives. All groups operated under the aegis of wider society, and concerns about problems such as national deterioration, the limits of state involvement in private lives or concerns about the permissive society impacted on maternity provision. Everyone involved in maternity was affected by the growing regulation of the experience, whether through education and training, the use of technology or the language of risks and right, normality and abnormality. Running through the century is the question of to whom did the experience of maternity actually belong? Mothers, midwives, doctors and society more broadly all at different times abrogated different elements of the experience for themselves, and put themselves at the centre of the stage.

Beyond this, the story of maternity in the twentieth century can perhaps best be regarded as the story of unintended consequences. Women campaigned, both collectively and individually, for the right to give birth in hospital with analgesia available for the birth, and several days' rest afterwards. What they got was often to be left alone in labour, and encouraged to accept interventions that they did not necessarily want or need. Similarly *Changing Childbirth* saw a broad professional and consumer consensus in favour of repositioning pregnancy and birth as physiological rather than pathological events. The sophisticated measures of risk designated to delineate the 'normal' and physiological from the 'abnormal' and pathological led inexorably to the pigeon-holing of certain pregnancies and births, and the rise in litigation by consumers increased the chances of defensive practice. Both of these issues saw the Caesarean section rate rising, at a time when all sides seemed to agree that it should be lowered.

Perhaps the answer to the vexed question of who controls childbirth is: everyone and no one. So many groups have a stake, and across the twentieth century different elements have held sway at different times, with regulation constraining the work and beliefs of all groups. Underlying this is the fact that women have continued to give birth, with the majority of babies delivered vaginally and with little intervention. Despite concerns about their role and professional status, midwives are still present at nearly all births and deliver about two-thirds of all babies; a proportion which has remained pretty constant across the period.

Further research into different aspects of maternity care would allow for a more nuanced understanding of beliefs and relationships. It would be interesting to look in more detail at relationships between professionals and women at a local level in order to explore patterns of care and belief. It would also be valuable to examine some of the marginalised voices in the story of maternity care: GPs, midwives who embraced technology, women who did not campaign for change, and obstetricians who supported a low-technology approach to pregnancy and birth. This book has only scratched the surface of the story of maternity in the twentieth century, but as an area that touches everyone's lives one way or another, it is hoped that it will stimulate further exploration and interpretation.

Appendix 1: Main government legislation relevant to maternity care

Midwives Act, 1902 [2 Edw. 7. c. 17]

The first midwives act, which covered England and Wales. It came into force in 1905, and included the creation of the Midwives Roll (an annually updated list of practising midwives), the creation of statutory supervision, the publication of Midwives Rules and sphere of practice, and minimum standards for the training and education of midwives. Central Midwives Board (CMB) created to oversee regulation, practice and supervision.

Notification of Births Act, 1907 [7 Edw. 7. c. 40]

An enabling act designed to improve assessment of birth rates and infant health through notification of a birth (after the 28th week of pregnancy) to the local Medical Officer of Health within 36 hours of it occurring. Births could be notified by midwives, doctors or fathers. The Health Department would then make arrangements for the infant to be visited by a Health Visitor.

National Insurance Act, 1911 [1 & 2 Geo. 5. c. 55]

Clauses relating to maternity gave the wives of men who paid National Insurance some maternity benefit.

Notification of Births Act (extension), 1915 [5 & 6 Geo. 5. c. 29]

This made the provisions of the 1907 Notification of Births Act compulsory across England and Wales.

Maternity and Child Welfare Act, 1918 [9 Geo. 5. c. 29]

An enabling act, giving legal recognition to maternal and child welfare services developed by local authorities, including health visitors, welfare clinics and mothercraft classes.

Midwives Act, 1918 [8 & 9 Geo. 5. c. 43]

Local authorities would now be responsible for fees and expenses paid to doctors called to maternity cases in an emergency (and could attempt to reclaim them from patients). Previously midwives had often ended up paying and struggling to reclaim fees from patients.

Midwives to be compensated for loss of earnings due to suspension from practice.

Ministry of Health Act, 1919 [9 & 10. Geo. 5. c. 21]

Abolished the Local Government Board, which oversaw all functions of local government after 1871.

The Ministry of Health was responsible for central government coordination of health issues, and several important Reports were published by them in the area of maternity care.

In 1968 the Ministry of Health was subsumed into the Department of Health and Social Security (DHSS), and became a separate Department of Health again in 1988.

Local Government Act, 1929 [19 Geo. 5. c. 17]

Transferred the functions of the Poor Law authorities (who ran workhouses and their associated infirmaries) to local councils. Many councils used their powers to develop the infirmaries as municipal hospitals and in-patient maternity provision and midwifery training was developed in these institutions. They were required to co-operate with voluntary hospitals to plan capacity and bed needs; a scheme which worked better in some areas than others.

An Act to Amend the Midwives Acts, 1902 to 1926, 1936 [26 Geo. 5 & 1 Edw. 8. c. 40]

All local authorities required to provide a salaried midwifery service, and to pay compensation to midwives who did not gain employment on surrender of their midwifery certificate. Salaried midwives were guaranteed time off, pensions and job security. They were provided with equipment and a uniform.

Midwives were no longer paid directly by women for care, although women were expected to pay the local authority.

Qualifications were developed under the Act for midwife teachers (the Midwife Teacher's Diploma or MTD), and for Supervisors of Midwives. All midwives now required to attend five-yearly refresher courses, and midwives returning to practice after a prolonged absence were required to complete a return to practice course.

Family Allowances Act, 1945 [8 & 9 Geo. 6. c. 41]

Children's allowances were proposed by the Beveridge Report. They could be claimed by either parent and gave an allowance of five shillings per week for every child after the first.

National Health Service Act, 1946 [9 & 10 Geo. 6. c. 81]

Took into national public ownership all hospitals, both local authority and voluntary.

Treatment and care were now free at the point of need, and the cost was covered out of general taxation.

GPs remained private and the NHS bought their services.

Maternity care now had a 'tripartite' structure. District midwives, welfare clinics and family planning were provided by local councils. Hospital care was provided by the NHS. GPs contracted to the NHS to provide maternity care.

Abortion Act, 1967 [1967 c. 87]

Private Members' Bill introduced by Liberal MP David Steel and supported by Labour government. Result of long campaigns for and against a change in the law. Abortion now legal under 28 weeks of pregnancy if agreed by two doctors that continuation of pregnancy would result in non-viable foetus, or would endanger physical or mental health of mothers. Health professionals entitled to express conscientious objection to giving routine care to women undergoing abortion.

Some doctors and some areas interpreted law very liberally, others very strictly.

National Health Service Reorganisation Act, 1973 [1973 c. 32]

Made provision for Area and Regional Health Authorities which now controlled all health-related activity, stripping local authorities of their remaining powers. Maternity services all now run by acute services, and employment of district midwives transferred to Regional Health Authorities. Family planning services and welfare clinics also now controlled by this umbrella group. Contraception now free.

Nurses, Midwives and Health Visitors Act, 1979 [1979 c. 36]

Abolished all the individual Boards which regulated nursing, midwifery and health visiting (including the CMB) and created the United Kingdom Central Council for Nursing, Midwifery and Health Visiting (known as the UKCC), with regional Board representation. Also created a single professional register with separate parts for those with different qualifications. UKCC started work in 1983.

The Human Fertilisation and Embryology Act, 1990 [1990 c. 37]

Reduced the time limit on abortions from 28 weeks of pregnancy to 24, although later abortions can be provided in exceptional circumstances.

Licensed and regulated fertility treatment clinics and the use of embryos and foetal cells for scientific research.

Nursing and Midwifery Order, 2001 [SI 2002/553]

Abolished UKCC and created Nursing and Midwifery Council (NMC) from April 2002. Covers nursing and midwifery and regulates training, education, regulation and the professional register.

Appendix 2: National reports relevant to maternity care

Government reports

Report of the Inter-departmental Committee on Physical Deterioration 1902

Set up as a result of concerns about the poor state of health of potential military recruits. Did not support fears of racial degeneration but drew attention to policies likely to ameliorate problems of poor diet, infant health, etc. Informed early ideas about state involvement in individual health.

Report of the Departmental Committee to Consider the Working of the Midwives Act 1902, 1909

Suggested that the Act was generally working well, that untrained midwives were a dying breed and that maternal mortality was falling in response to the Act.

Report on the Future Provision of Medical and Allied Services (Dawson Report) 1920

One of the founding documents of the National Health Service because it suggested a national system of health care based around the General Practitioner and the Primary Health Centre, backed up by secondary hospital services. It argued that preventative medicine, including midwifery services, was as important as curative services.

Final Report of the Departmental Committee on Maternal Mortality and Morbidity 1932

Followed the Interim Report of 1930. Both suggested that a large proportion of maternal mortality was preventable, and suggested that more antenatal care and more hospital beds for maternity cases were required.

Report on an Investigation into Maternal Mortality 1937

Tried to play down extent to which maternal deaths were preventable, as it was feared that earlier reports had increased public anxiety about why deaths were not being prevented. It emphasised individual clinical factors over social or economic ones.

Report of the Inter-departmental Committee on Abortion (Birkett Report) 1939

Set up after the 1937 Maternal Mortality Report which suggested that the illegal abortion rate was rising and was contributing to maternal mortality. The Report decided that numbers of abortions were almost impossible to estimate, but that the rate seemed to be rising and the law against abortion should be better applied. The Report was published just as the Second World War broke out and so was never acted upon.

Report on Social Insurance and Allied Services (Beveridge Report) 1942

A best seller, particularly among the Army, because it held out the promise of a better world after the Depression of the 1930s and the Second World War. It called for comprehensive health services, social security, children's allowances and the maintenance of full employment, all covered by general taxation and National Insurance. These aims were broadly accepted by successive Labour and Conservative governments and laid the foundations of the Welfare State and the NHS.

Report of Midwives Salaries Committee (Rushcliffe Report) 1943

Set up to look at midwifery salaries, but also made wide-ranging recommendations covering off duty, the provision of uniforms and other facilities. Called for the role of midwife to be accorded more respect by society.

Royal Commission on Population Report 1949

Wide-ranging Report which considered the falling birth rate and its implications. Looked at birth control, expectations of families and of women, and of standards of living. Considered how motherhood might be made more attractive to women through the provision of nurseries, home helps and amelioration of cost of child rearing.

Report of the Working Party on Midwives (Stocks Report) 1949

Considered the shortage of midwives and their conditions of work. Called for midwives to be as respected as doctors and teachers. Suggested that midwifery education should be subsumed into that of nurses.

Report of the Committee on the Cost of the National Health Service (Guillebaud Report) 1956

Set up in response to concerns that the NHS was spending money like water, and was unaffordable. Report suggested that, in fact, the NHS was providing good value for money. It did claim that the Maternity Services were 'in a state of some confusion' however, a statement which led to the creation of the Cranbrook Committee to consider this point.

Report of the Maternity Services Committee (Cranbrook Report) 1959

Set up to explore the structure of the Maternity Services after comments by the Guillebaud Committee. Decided that the tripartite system of organisation (GPs, local authorities, hospitals) worked reasonably well, and did not recommend its dismantling.

The Report noted that the rate of hospital births was increasing, and called for hospital beds to be available for 75 per cent of maternities. Called for domiciliary births to continue to be supported by staff and revenue.

Central Health Services Council Standing Maternity and Midwifery Advisory Committee: Human Relations in Obstetrics 1961

Suggested that hospital-based maternity care should be 'humanised' in order to give women a better experience. Drew on women's concerns about the cattle market aspect of antenatal clinics, for example.

Committee on Senior Nursing Staff Structure (Salmon Report) 1966

Looked at the structure and pay of nursing and midwifery hospital management and developed different managerial grades up to Chief Nursing Officer. Abolished post of hospital Matron (became Nursing Officer). The office of Matron was re-established after 2001.

Domiciliary Midwifery and Maternity Bed Needs (Peel Report) 1970

Called for hospital maternity beds to be available for all women, on the grounds that hospital birth was safer than home birth.

Report of the Committee on Nursing (Briggs Report) 1972

Looked at the training of nurses and midwives, and made calls for them to become research aware and research active. Suggested the creation of a nationwide regulatory body (which was created as the UKCC 1983).

Second Report from the Social Services Committee: Perinatal and Neonatal Mortality (Short Report) 1980

Report called for GP maternity units to be phased out on the grounds of safety. Just stopped short of calling for home birth to be outlawed. Noted that midwives were often not using their full range of skills, and called for them to be seen as an integral part of the maternity team.

Working Group on Inequalities in Health (Black Report) 1980

A report commissioned by the Labour government in 1977, whose conclusions were largely rejected by the incumbent Conservative government when it was published. It suggested that wide social class disparities in health and life expectancy persisted, and had in some areas increased, despite over 30 years of the NHS.

First Report of the Maternity Services Advisory Committee: Maternity Care in Action. Part 1 – Antenatal Care 1982

Second Report of the Maternity Services Advisory Committee: Maternity Care in Action. Part 2 – Care during Childbirth 1984

Third Report of the Maternity Services Advisory Committee: Maternity Care in Action. Part 3 – Care of the Mother and Baby 1985

A series of reports which aimed to put the recommendations of the Short Report into action. They described themselves as 'a guide to good practice and a plan for action'. Their recommendations were largely based on advice rather than research evidence.

Report of the Committee of Enquiry into Human Fertilisation and Embryology (Warnock Report) 1984

First 'test tube baby' born in 1978. Committee called for licensing and regulation around research and clinical procedures, with a named regulator. Noted the 'special status' of the embryo, which had no rights of ownership over it. Called for counselling for couples prior to fertility treatment and the right of children so born to have basic information about their background from the age of 18.

Report of the Committee of Inquiry into the Future Development of the Public Health Function (Acheson Report) 1988

Focused on public health as a way of tackling health inequalities. Supported intervention around infant feeding, maternal obesity and smoking as well as broader health issues across the life cycle.

Health Committee Second Report: Maternity Services (Winterton Report) 1992

Looked at the structure of the maternity services, and took evidence from a range of interested parties including the NCT and AIMS as well as midwives and doctors. The government did not initially accept its recommendations, but it was widely heralded by midwives and women's groups for putting women at the heart of maternity care, and for enshrining ideas of choice and control continuity for women.

The Report suggested that the medical model of maternity care was largely unproven and that to encourage all women to give birth in hospital on the grounds of safety was wrong.

Report of the Expert Maternity Group: Changing Childbirth (Cumberlege Report) 1993

Built on the work of the Winterton Report by surveying best practice in the maternity services, and creating targets for change with a five-year time limit (for example, that every woman should have a named midwife, and that at least 75 per cent of women should know the person who cares for them during labour).

Report by the Standing Nursing and Midwifery Advisory Committee Midwifery: Delivering our Future 1998

Report explored role of midwife following *Changing Childbirth*, in order to deliver 'woman focused care'. Suggested midwives needed to 're-skill' through education, research and the development of autonomous practice.

Making a Difference: Strengthening the Nursing, Midwifery and Health Visiting Contribution to Health and Healthcare 1999

Explored how nursing, midwifery and health visiting could contribute to the 'new' NHS, and rising consumer expectations. Established consultant posts for the three professions, set up groups to develop 'national quality standards', and planned to replace UKCC with a new body. Midwives encouraged to take on greater public health role.

Interest group reports

Joint Committee of the Royal College of Obstetricians and Gynaecologists and the Population Investigation Committee (1948) Maternity in Great Britain, Oxford University Press

Looked at the social and economic aspects of pregnancy and birth, through questionnaires administered through health visitors to women who delivered 3–8 March 1946. It looked at antenatal, intra-partum and postnatal care, as well as pain relief, infant feeding and the costs of childrearing among other topics.

The 1958 Perinatal Mortality Survey (Butler and Bonham 1963)

Research carried out under the auspices of the NBTF, used similar survey method to that of the 1948 Report above, to study all births which occurred 4–9 March 1958. Results and discussion were skewed towards perinatal mortality, but the Report contained other details including the use of pain relief and the professional in attendance at delivery.

The Report had a significant impact on maternity service policy in the1960s, but its analysis has been critiqued by Tew (1990).

British Births 1970

A joint venture between the NBTF and RCOG, designed to build on the results 1958 Survey, by studying all births from 5–10 April 1970. It focused on perinatal mortality (Report published 1978) and on the first week of life (Report published 1975). The analysis from this Survey informed maternity service policy, but has been critiqued by Tew (1990).

Audit Commission First Class Delivery: Improving Maternity Services in England and Wales 1997

First large-scale audit of maternity services following *Changing Childbirth*. Found women generally pleased with their care, although most dissatisfaction around postnatal care.

Social Exclusion Unit: Teenage Pregnancy 1999

Set out ten-year plan for reducing teenage pregnancy rates by 50 per cent, focusing on teenagers from lower social economic groups.

The National Sentinel Caesarean Section Audit Report (2001) (Paranjothy and Thomas)

An audit jointly developed by RCOG, RCM and NCT and the Royal College of Anaesthetists to explore the reasons for the rising Caesarean section rate (21.5 per cent in 2000–1, up from 9 per cent in 1980). A one-day conference which followed on from the Report suggested actions to reduce the rate, including more one-to-one care, and encouraging women to stay at home longer when in early labour.

Confidential Enquiries into Maternal Deaths

These reports were first commissioned in the 1930s following concerns about maternal mortality rates. An outline of their results was initially published within the Annual Reports of the Chief Medical Officer until 1951. Thereafter they were collated as a separate document. They have always been produced triennially with the intention of exploring and learning lessons from every maternal death. The enquiries and reports have, until relatively recently, been in the hands of members of RCOG.

Bibliography

Primary sources

Collection of oral history interviews conducted and held by Tania McIntosh
Collection of oral history interviews held by Nottingham City Council Local
    Studies Library

    British Journal of Midwifery
    The British Medical Journal (*BMJ*)
    The Guardian and *Manchester Guardian* newspaper
    The Independent newspaper
    Jessop Hospital for Women Annual Reports
    Journal of the Royal Sanitary Institute
    The Lancet
    LGB Annual Reports 1900–18
    Medical Officer of Health Reports Nottingham
    Medical Officer of Health Reports Sheffield
    Midwifery
    Midwifery Matters (www.midwifery.org)
    Midwives Chronicle and Nursing Notes
    Ministry of Health Annual Reports
    Modern Midwife
    NCT Annual Reports
    The Observer newspaper
    Public Health 1927
    Research and the Midwife Conference Proceedings
    Sheffield Independent newspaper
    Sheffield and Rotherham Independent
    Sheffield Royal Infirmary Annual Reports
    Sheffield Telegraph newspaper
    The Times newspaper

Secondary sources

Addison, P. (1975) *The road to 1945: British politics and the Second World War*,
    London: Cape.

Allison, J. (1994) 'Place of birth: finding the next step forward', in Chamberlain, G. and Patel, N. (1994) *The Future of the Maternity Services*, London: RCOG Press.
——(1996) *Delivered at Home*, London: Chapman & Hall.
Allotey, J. (2007) 'Discourses on the function of the pelvis in childbearing: ancient times until the present day', unpublished thesis, University of Sheffield.
Allotey, J.C. and McIntosh, T. (2009) 'History of midwifery: professional luxury or essential legacy', *MIDIRS*, 19(4), 488–91.
Anderson, T. (1995) 'Empowering women to make informed choice', *Midwifery Matters*, Issue 67.
——(2006) 'MIDIRS midwifery digest', *MIDIRS*, 16(2), 279–81.
Apple, R.D. (1995) 'Constructing mothers: scientific motherhood in the nineteenth and twentieth centuries', *Social History of Medicine*, 8, 161–78.
ARM (1985) 'The Vision', in *Radical Midwifery: Celebrating 21 Years of A.R.M.*, Ormskirk: Association of Radical Midwives.
——(2000) *Vision for Midwifery Education*, Ormskirk: Association of Radical Midwives.
Arney, W.R. (1982) *Power and the Profession of Obstetrics*, Chicago: University of Chicago Press.
Ashton, R. (1992) 'Committed to caring, committed to change', *Midwives Chronicle and Nursing Notes*, May: 106–7.
Aspinall, K., Nelson, B., Patterson, T. and Sims, A. (1997) *An Extraordinary Woman: The Story of Ann Garner, A Sheffield Midwife*, Sheffield: Ann's Trust Fund.
Aveling, J.H. (1872, reprinted 1967) *English Midwives: Their History and Prospects*, London: Hugh K. Elliott Ltd.
Bailey, R.E. (1972) *Mayes' Midwifery*, London: Baillière Tindall.
Bailey, R.E. (1976) *Mayes' Midwifery: A Textbook for Midwives*, London: Baillière Tindall.
Balaskas, J. (1991) *New Active Birth: A Concise Guide to Natural Childbirth*, London: Thorsons.
Balaskas, J. and Gordon, Y. (1992) *Water Birth: The Concise Guide to Using Water during Pregnancy, Birth and Infancy*, London: Thorsons.
Ball, J.A., Flint, C., Garvey, M., Jackson-Baker, A. and Page, L. (1992) *Who's Left Holding the Baby? An organisational framework for making the most of Midwifery Services*, Leeds: Nuffield Institute.
Ballantyne, J.W. (1901) 'Pro-maternity care', *British Medical Journal*, i, 813.
——(1914) *Expectant Motherhood: It's Supervision and Hygiene*, London: Cassell & Company.
Barbour, R.S. (1990) 'Fathers: the emergence of a new consumer group' in Garcia, J., Kilpatrick, R. and Richards, M. (eds) (1990) *The Politics of Maternity Care: Services for Childbearing Women in Twentieth-Century Britain*, Oxford: Clarendon Press.
Beech, B.L. (1992) 'Rights and wrongs in maternity care', *Modern Midwife*, 1, 8–10.
Beech, B.L. and Robinson J. (1996) *Ultrasound? Unsound*, London: AIMS.
Beech, B.L. and Willington, S. (2007) 'Listen With Mother', *AIMS Journal*, 19(2).
Beinart, J. (1990) 'Obstetric analgesia and the control of childbirth in twentieth-century Britain', in Garcia, J., Kilpatrick, R. and Richards, M. (1990) *The politics of maternity care*, Oxford: Clarendon Press.
Bell, F. (1907, reprinted 1985) *At the Works: A Study of a Manufacturing Town*, London: Virago Press.
Bell, R.E. (1934) 'Maternal mortality in Liverpool', *Public Health*, 47, 330–34.

Benoit, C., Wrede, S., Bourgeault, I., Sandall, J., De Vries, R. and van Teijlingen, E.R. (2005) 'Understanding the social organisation of maternity care systems: midwifery as a touchstone', *Sociology of Health and Illness*, 27(6), 722–37.

Berkeley, C. (1926) 'Save the women and children', *British Medical Journal*, i, 4–8.

Berridge, V. (ed.) (2005) *Making Health Policy: Networks in Research and Policy after 1945*, Amsterdam: Rodopi.

——(2008) 'History matters? History's role in health policy making', *Medical History*, 52(3), 311–26.

Berridge, V., Christie, D.A. and Tansey, E.M. (eds) (2006) *Public health in the 1980s and 1990s: decline and rise?* Wellcome Witnesses to Twentieth Century Medicine. Volume 26, London: The Wellcome Trust.

Birdwood, G.T. (1932) *Advice to the Expectant Mother: Fifty Antenatal Talks. For the use of doctors, nurses and expectant mothers.* London: John Bale, Sons and Danielsson Ltd.

BirthChoiceUK (2012) *Historical caesarean rates*, http://www.birthchoiceuk.com/Professionals/CSHistory.htm. Accessed 11.01.2012.

Blodgett, H. (1989) *Centuries of Female Days: English Women's Private Diaries*, Gloucester: Alan Sutton Publishing.

Blom, P. (2008) *The Vertigo Years: Change and Culture in the West, 1900–1914*, London: Weidenfeld and Nicholson.

Bock, G. and Thane, P. (eds) (1991) *Maternity and Gender Policies: Women and the Rise of European Welfare States, 1880s–1950s*, London: Routledge.

Bonney, V. (1919) 'The continuing high maternal mortality of child-bearing: the reason and the remedy', *Proceedings of the Royal Society for Medicine*, 12, 75–107.

Bornat, J., Perks, R. and Thompson, P. (1999) *Oral history health and welfare*, London: Routledge.

Borsay, A. and Hunter, B. (eds) (forthcoming: 2012) *Nursing and Midwifery in Britain Since 1700*, Basingstoke: Palgrave Macmillan.

Borst, C.G. (1988) 'The training and practise of midwives: a Wisconsin study', *Bulletin of the History of Medicine*, 62, 606–27.

——(1995) *Catching Babies: The Professionalisation of Childbirth, 1870–1920*, London: Harvard University Press.

Bourgeault, I.L. (2006) *Push! The Struggle for Midwifery in Ontario*, Quebec: McGill-Queens University Press.

Bourgeault, I.L., Benoit, C. and Davis-Floyd, R. (2004) *Reconceiving midwifery*, Quebec: McGill-Queens Press.

Bourne, G. (1989) *Pregnancy*, London: Pan Books Ltd.

Bradley, S., Robinson, S. and Golden, J. (1981) 'A preliminary report on the research project on the role and responsibilities of the midwife: Part 2', *Midwives Chronicle*, 94, 49–53.

Brain, M. (1991) 'The place of women in the NHS', *Midwives Chronicle*, 104, 343–46.

Browne, F.W.S., Ludovici, A.M. and Roberts, H. (eds) (1935) *Abortion*, London: Allen and Unwin.

——(1935) 'The right to abortion' in Browne, F.W.S., Ludovici, A.M. and Roberts, H. (eds) (1935) *Abortion*, London: Allen and Unwin.

Bullough, L.A. (1917) 'Midwifery service in the West Riding administrative area', *Public Health*, 31, 126–32.

Burtch, B. (1994) *Trials of Labour: The Re-emergence of Midwifery*, Quebec: McGill-Queens University Press.

Butler, N.R. and Bonham, D.G. (1963) *Perinatal Mortality: The First Report of the 1958 British Perinatal Mortality Survey, under the auspices of The National Birthday Trust Fund*, London: E. & S. Livingstone Ltd.

Butterfield, H. (1931) *The Whig Interpretation of History*, London: G. Bell and Sons.

Cahill, H.A. (2001) 'Male appropriation and medicalization of childbirth: an historical analysis', *Journal of Advanced Nursing*, 33(3), 334–42.

Cairns, A. (ed.) (2006) *Home Births: Stories to Inspire and Inform*, Gloucestershire: Lonely Scribe.

Cameron, J. and Ellwood, D. (2006) 'Risk perception and analysis in Australia' **in** Symon, A. (ed.) (2006) *Risk and Choice in Maternity Care: An international perspective*, Edinburgh: Elsevier.

Campbell, J.M. (1923) *The training of midwives, Ministry of Health Reports on Health and other Subjects*, London: HMSO.

——(1924) *Maternal Mortality*, London: HMSO.

——(1927) *The Protection of Motherhood*, London: HMSO.

——(1935) *Maternity Services*, London: HMSO.

Campbell, J.M., Cameron, I.D. and Jones, D.M. (1932) *High Maternal Mortality in Certain Areas*, London: HMSO.

Campbell, N., Harvey, D. and Norman, A.P. (1975) 'Increased frequency of neonatal jaundice in a maternity hospital', *British Medical Journal*, 2, 548–52.

Campbell, R. and Macfarlane, A. (1990) 'Recent debate on the place of birth' **in** Garcia, J., Kilpatrick, R. and Richards, M. (eds) (1990) *The Politics of Maternity Care: Services for Childbearing Women in Twentieth-Century Britain*, Oxford: Clarendon Press.

Carpenter, M. (1977) 'The new managerialism and professionalism in nursing' **in** Stacey, M., Reid, M., Heath, C. and Dingwall, R. (eds) (1977) *Health and the Division of Labour*, London: Croom Helm.

Carr, E.H. (1961, reprinted 1981) *What is History?*, Harmondsworth: Pelican Books.

Carter, G. (1948) *The Midwives Dictionary and Encyclopaedia*, London: Faber and Faber Ltd.

Cartwright, A. (1964) *Human Relations and Hospital Care*, London: Routledge and Kegan Paul.

——(1979) *The Dignity of Labour? A Study of Childbearing and Induction*, London: Tavistock Publications Limited.

Cassie, E. (1929) 'Maternal mortality and allied problems', *Public Health*, 42, 329–33.

Chalmers, I., Enkin, M. and Keirse, M.J.N.C. (1989) *Effective care in pregnancy and childbirth*, Oxford: Oxford University Press.

Chamberlain, G. and Patel, N. (1994) *The Future of the Maternity Services*, London: RCOG Press.

Christie, D.A and Tansey, E.M. (eds) (2001) *Maternal Care*. Wellcome Witnesses to Twentieth Century Medicine. Volume 12, London: The Wellcome Trust.

Clark, A. (1919) *Working Life of Women in the Seventeenth Century*, London: Routledge & Sons.

Clark, E. (2000) 'The historical context of research in midwifery' **in** Procter, S. and Renfrew, M. (eds) (2000) *Linking research and practice in midwifery*, London: Baillière Tindall.

Colebrook, L. (1926) 'Some laboratory investigations in connection with puerperal fever', *Proceedings of the Royal Society for Medicine*, 19:31–42.

Colebrook, L. (1956) 'The story of puerperal fever – 1800 to 1950', *British Medical Journal*, i, 247–52.

Colebrook, L. and Kenny, M. (1936) 'Treatment with Prontosil of puerperal infections due to haemolytic streptococci', *The Lancet*, ii, 1319–22.

Collings, J.S. (1950) 'General practice in England today: a reconnaissance', *The Lancet*, i: 555–85.

Cookson, I. (1954) 'Domiciliary obstetrics', *British Medical Journal*, 1, 841.

Coulter, A. (2002) *The Autonomous Patient: Ending Paternalism in Medical Care*, London: Nuffield Trust.

Crawford, M.D. (1932) 'The obstetric forceps and its use', *The Lancet*, i, 1239–43.

Curtis, P., Ball, L. and Kirkham, M. (2006) 'Why do midwives leave? (Not) being the kind of midwife you want to be', *British Journal of Midwifery*, 14(1), 27–31.

Curzon, P. and Mountrose, U.M. (1976) 'The general practitioners role in the management of labour', *British Medical Journal*, 2, 1433–4.

Dale, P. and Fisher, K. (2009) 'Implementing the 1902 Midwives Act: assessing problems, developing services and creating a new role for a variety of female practitioners', *Women's History Review*, 18(3), 427–52.

Dangerfield, G. (1935, reprinted 1983) *The Strange Death of Liberal England*, St Albans: Paladin.

Davies, C. (ed.) (1980) *Re-writing Nursing History*, London: Croom Helm.

Davies, C. (1988) 'The Health Visitor as mother's friend: a woman's place in public health 1900–914', *Social History of Medicine*, 1, 39–59.

Davin, A. (1978) 'Imperialism and motherhood', *History Workshop Journal*, 5, 9–65.

Davis, A. (2007) 'Motherhood in Oxfordshire c. 1945–70: A study of attitudes, experiences and ideals', unpublished thesis, University of Oxford.

——(2011) 'A revolution in maternity care? Women and the maternity services, Oxfordshire c. 1948–74', *Social History of Medicine*, doi: 10.1093/shm/hkq092.

——(forthcoming: 2012) *Modern Motherhood: Women and Family in England c.1945–2000*, Manchester: Manchester University Press.

Dawson, Lord (1920) 'Medicine and the state', *British Medical Journal*, i, 743–45.

De Brouwere, V., Tonglet, R. and Van Lerberghe, W. (2002) 'Strategies for reducing maternal mortality in developing countries: what can we learn from the history of the industrialized West?', *Tropical Medicine and International Health*, 3(10), 771–82.

Dent, M. and Whitehead, S. (2003) *Managing Professional Identities: Knowledge, Performativities, and the 'New' Professional*, London: Routledge.

Devlin, V. (ed.) (1995) *Motherhood: from 1920 to the Present Day*, Edinburgh: Polygon.

Dick-Read, G. (1933, reprinted 2004) *Natural Childbirth*, London: Pinter and Martin.

——(1942) *Revelation of Childbirth*, London: William Heinemann.

Dike, P. (2005) 'Student midwives: views of the direct entry programme', *Midwives*, 8(7), 314–17.

DOH (1993) *A Study of Midwife- and GP-led Maternity Units*, London: NHS Management Executive.

——(1993) *A Vision for the Future: The Nursing, Midwifery and Health Visiting Contribution to Health and Health Care*, London: NHS Management Executive.

Donald, A. (1894) *An Introduction to Midwifery: A Handbook for Medical Students and Midwives*, London: Charles Griffin and Company, Ltd.

Donald, I. (1964) *Practical Obstetric Problems*, 3rd edn, London: Lloyd-Luke (Medical Books) Ltd.

——(1972) *Practical Obstetric Problems*, 4th edn, London: Lloyd-Luke (Medical Books) Ltd.

——(1979) *Practical Obstetric Problems*, 5th edn, London: Lloyd-Luke (Medical Books) Ltd.

Donnison, J. (1988) *Midwives and Medical Men: A History of The Struggle for the Control of Childbirth*, 2nd edn, London: Historical Publications.

Donzelot, J. (1979) *The Policing of Families*, Pantheon Books: London.

Dove, I. (1985) 'Powerful and peripheral: A history of Alice Gregory, Leila Parnell and Maud Cashmore, founders of the British Hospital for Mothers and Babies, Woolwich, and the National Training School for Midwives', unpublished dissertation, University of Kent.

Dowling, S. (1984) 'The provision of community antenatal services', **in** Zander, L. and Chamberlain, G. (eds) (1984) *Pregnancy care for the 1990s*, London: The Royal Society of Medicine and the Macmillan Press.

Drife, J. (2002) 'The start of life: a history of obstetrics', *Post Graduate Medical Journal*, 78, 311–15.

Durward, L. and Evans, R. (1990) 'Pressure groups and maternity care' **in** Garcia, J., Kilpatrick, R. and Richards, M. (eds) (1990) *The Politics of Maternity Care: Services for Childbearing Women in Twentieth-Century Britain*, Oxford: Clarendon Press.

Dwork, D. (1987) *War is Good for Babies and Other Young Children: A History of the Infant and Child Welfare Movement in England 1898–1918*, London: Tavistock Routledge.

Dye, N.S. (1986–87) 'Modern obstetrics and working class women: the New York Midwifery Dispensary, 1890–1920', *Journal of Social History*, 20, 549–64.

Ehrenreich, B. and English, D. (1976) *Witches, Midwives and Nurses: A History of Women Healers*, New York: The City of New York University Press.

——(1979) *For Her Own Good: 150 Years of the Experts Advice to Women*, New York: Anchor.

Enkin, M., Keirse, M.J.N.C. and Chambers, I. (1991) *A Guide to Effective Care in Pregnancy and Childbirth*, Oxford: Oxford University Press.

Enkin, M.W., Keirse, M.J.N.C., Renfrew, M.J. and Neilson, J.P. (1995) *A guide to effective care in pregnancy and childbirth*, 2nd edn, Oxford: Oxford University Press.

Etzioni, A. (ed.) (1969) *The Semi-Professions and Their Organization*, New York: Free Press.

Eustance, A. (2000) 'A life in midwifery', *Midwifery Matters*, Issue 59.

Fairbairn, J.S. (1914) *A textbook for midwives*, Oxford: Oxford University Press.

——(1931) 'The medical and psychological aspects of gynaecology', *The Lancet*, ii, 999–1004.

Fannin, M. (2006) 'Global midwifery and the technologies of emotion', *ACME: An International E-journal for Critical Geographies*, 5(1), 70–88.

Farrell, L.A. (1979) 'The history of eugenics: a bibliographical review', *Annals of Science*, 36, 111–23.

Fealy, G.M. (ed.) (2005) *Care to Remember: Nursing and Midwifery in Ireland*, Cork: Mercier Press.

Fildes, V., Marks, L. and Marland, H. (1992) *Women and Children First: International Maternal and Infant Welfare,1870–1945*, London: Routledge.

Finch, J. (1982) 'The maternity defence fund. Litigation: a simple step forward', *Nursing Mirror*, 155(10), 15.

Fisher, K. (2008) *Birth Control, Sex, and Marriage in Britain 1918–1960*, Oxford: Oxford University Press.

Fissell, M.E. (2003) 'Hairy women and naked truths: gender and the politics of knowledge in Aristotle's Masterpiece', *William and Mary Quarterly*, 60(1), 43–74.

Fleming, V.E.M. (1998) 'Autonomous or automatons? An exploration through the history of the concept of autonomy in midwifery in Scotland and New Zealand', *Nursing Ethics*, 5, 43–51.

Flint, C. (1993) *Midwifery Teams and Caseloads*, Oxford: Butterworth-Heinemann.

Flynn, A.M., Kelly, J., Hollins, G. and Lynch, P.F. (1978) 'Ambulation in labour', *British Medical Journal*, 2, 591–93.

Forbes, T.R. (1966) *The midwife and the witch*, Newhaven: Yale University Press.

——(1962) 'Midwifery and witchcraft', *Journal of the History of Medicine*, 17, 264–93.

Foucault, M. (1963, reprinted (English translation) in 2003) *The Birth of the Clinic*, London: Routledge Classics.

Fox, E. (1991) 'Powers of life and death: aspects of maternal welfare in England and Wales between the wars', *Social History of Medicine*, 35, 328–52.

——(1993) 'An honourable calling or a despised occupation: licensed midwifery and its relation to district nursing in England and Wales before 1948', *Social History of Medicine*, 6, 237–59.

——(1994) 'District nursing in England and Wales before the National Health Service: the neglected evidence', *Medical History*, 38, 303–21.

——(1996) 'Universal health care and self-help: paying for district nursing before the National Health Service', *Twentieth Century British History*, 7(1), 83–109.

Francombe, C., Savage, W., Churchill, H. and Lewison, H. (1993) *Caesarean Birth in Britain*, London: Middlesex University Press.

Fraser, D. (2003) *The Evolution of the British Welfare State: A History of Social Policy since the Industrial Revolution*, Basingstoke: Palgrave Macmillan.

Garcia, J., Garforth, S. and Ayers, S. (1985) 'Midwives confined? Labour ward policies and routines', *Research and the Midwife Conference Proceedings 1985*, 1–30.

Garcia, J., Kilpatrick, R. and Richards, M. (eds) (1990) *The Politics of Maternity Care: Services for Childbearing Women in Twentieth-Century Britain*, Oxford: Clarendon Press.

Garland Collins, F. (1934) 'A midwife as a carrier of infection', *The Lancet*, ii, 718.

Garrett, W.J. and Robinson, D.E. (1970) *Ultrasound in Clinical Obstetrics*, Illinois: Charles C. Thomas.

Gaskin, I.M. (1975) *Spiritual Midwifery*, Summertown: Book Publishing Co.

Geddes, G. (1926) *Puerperal Septicaemia: its Causation, Symptoms, Prevention and Treatment*, Bristol: Wright.

Ghosh, A. and Hudson, F.P. (1972) 'Oxytocic agents and neonatal hyperbilirubinaemia', *The Lancet*, ii, 823.

Gifford, K.-A. (1996) 'Changing Childbirth in Nottingham', *Midwifery Matters*, Issue 71.

Glennerster, H. (2007) *British social policy 1945 to the present*, Oxford: Blackwell.

Graham, I.D. (1997) *Episiotomy: Challenging Obstetric Interventions*, London: Blackwell Science Ltd.

Granshaw, L. (1989) '"Fame and fortune by means of bricks and mortar": the medical profession and specialist hospitals in Britain, 1800–1948', in Granshaw, L. and Porter, R. (eds) (1989) *The Hospital in History*, London: Routledge.

Granshaw, L. and Porter, R. (eds) (1989) *The Hospital in History*, London: Routledge.

Grant, J. (1981) 'Research and the Midwife Conference', *Midwifery Matters*, Issue 9.

Green, J.M., Coupland, V.A. and Kitzinger, J.V. (1998) *Great Expectations: a Prospective Study of Women's Expectations and Experiences of Childbirth*, Hale: Books for Midwives.

Greer, G. (1971) *The Female Eunuch*, London: Paladin Grafton Books.

Guyatt, G. (1992) 'Evidence based medicine: a new approach to teaching the practice of medicine', *Journal of the American Medical Association*, 268(17), 2420–25.

Hadfield, S.J. (1953) 'A field survey of General Practice, 1951–52', *British Medical Journal*, 2, 683–706.

Hall, L.A. (1997) '"I have never met the normal women": Stella Browne and the politics of womanhood', *Women's History Review*, 6(2), 157–82.

——(2011) *The life and times of Stella Browne: feminist and free spirit*, London: IB Tauris.

Hannah, M.E., Hannah, W.J., Hewson, S.A., Saigal, S. and Willan, A.R. *et al.* (2000) 'Planned caesarean section versus planned vaginal birth for breech presentation at term: a randomized multicentre trial. Term Breech Trial Collaborative Group', *The Lancet*, 356, 1375–83.

Hannam, J. (1997) *Rosalind Paget: The Midwife, The Women's Movement and Reform Before 1914* in Marland, H. and Rafferty, A.M. (eds) (1997) *Midwives, Society and Childbirth: Debates and Controversies in the Modern Period*, London: Routledge.

Hanson, C. (2003) 'Save the Mothers? Representations of pregnancy in the 1930s', *Literature and History*, 12(2), 51–61.

——(2004) *A Cultural History of Pregnancy: Pregnancy, Medicine and Culture in Britain, 1750–2000*, Basingstoke: Palgrave Macmillan.

Hardyment, C. (2007) *Dream Babies: Childcare advice from John Locke to Gina Ford*, London: Jonathan Cape.

Harley, D. (1990) 'Historians as demonologists: The myth of the midwife-witch', *Social History of Medicine*, 3(1), 1–26.

——(1993) 'Provincial midwives in England: Lancashire and Cheshire', in Marland, H. (ed.) (1993) *The Art of Midwifery: Early Modern Midwives in Europe*, London: Routledge.

Harvey, H.G. (1950) 'The GP and the maternity service', *British Medical Journal*, 1, 903.

Heagerty, B.V. (1990) 'Gender and professionalisation: the struggle for British Midwifery, 1900–936', unpublished thesis, Michigan State University.

——(1996) 'Reassessing the guilty: The Midwives Act and the control of English midwives in the early twentieth century' in Kirkham, M. (ed.) (1996) *Supervision of Midwives*, Hale: Books for Midwives Press.

——(1997) 'Willing hand maidens of science? The struggle over the new midwife in early twentieth century England' in Kirkham, M.J. and Perkins, E.R. (eds) (1997) *Reflections on Midwifery*, London: Baillière Tindall.

Heardman, H. (1951) *Relaxation and exercises for natural childbirth*, London: E&S Livingstone.

Henderson, C. (1984) 'Influences and interactions surrounding the midwife's decision to rupture the membranes', *Research and the Midwife Conference Proceedings 1984*, 68–85.

Hicks, C. (1992) 'Research in midwifery: are midwives their own worst enemies?', *Midwifery*, 8, 12–18.

Hicks, J. and Allen, G. (1999) *A Century of Change: Trends in UK statistics since 1900*, London: House of Commons Research Paper.

Hine, D.C. (2005) *Black Women in White: Racial Conflict and Cooperation in the Nursing Profession, 1890–1950*, Bloomington: Indiana University Press.

HM Govt. (1904) *Report of Inter-departmental Committee on Physical Deterioration*, vol 1–3, xxxii, cd 2175, London.

Hobby, E. (ed.) (1999) *The Midwives Book: Or the Whole Art of Midwifry Discovered by Jane Sharp*, Oxford: Oxford University Press.

Howat, R.D. (1922) *The Threshold of Motherhood: A Handbook for the Pregnant Woman*, Glasgow: Maclehouse, Jackson and Co.

Humphries, S. and Gordon, P. (1993) *A Labour of Love: The Experience of Parenthood in Britain 1900–1950*, London: Sidgwick and Jackson.

Illingworth, R.S. (1953) *The Normal Child: Some Problems of the First Three Years and their Treatment*, London: J. & A. Churchill Ltd.

Inch, S. (1982) *Birthrights*, London: Hutchinson.

Jalland, P. (1988) *Women, Marriage and Politics 1860–1914*, Oxford: Oxford University Press.

James, D.W. (1950) 'The General Practitioner and the Maternity Service', *British Medical Journal*, 1, 598–602.

Johnson, T.J. (1972) *Professions and Power*, London: Macmillan.

Johnstone, R.W. (1949) *The Midwives Text-Book of the Principles and Practice of Midwifery*, London: Adam and Charles Black.

Jones, G. (1980) *Social Darwinism and English Thought*, Sussex: Harvester Press.

Jowitt, M. (1998) 'Changing Childbirth: the continuing challenge', *Midwifery Matters*, Issue 77.

Kargar, I. (1996) 'MIDIRS is 10 years old: how it began' *Midwifery Matters*, Issue 69, 16.

Kennedy, G.L. (1957) 'Domiciliary midwifery', *British Medical Journal*, 2, 1216–19.

King, H. (1993) 'The politick midwife: models of midwifery in the work of Elizabeth Cellier' **in** Marland, H. (ed.) (1993) *The Art of Midwifery: Early Modern Midwives in Europe*, London: Routledge.

——(2007) *Midwifery, Obstetrics and the Rise of Gynaecology*, London: Ashgate.

Kirchmeier, R. (1984) 'Influences on mothers' reactions to caesarean birth', *Research and the Midwife Conference Proceedings 1984*, 86–101.

Kirkham, M. (1981) 'Midwives and research', *Midwifery Matters*, Issue 10.

——(1989) 'Midwives and information-giving during labour', **in** Robinson, S. and Thomson, A.M. (eds) (1989) *Midwives, Research and Childbirth: Volume 1*, London: Chapman and Hall.

——(1996) 'Introduction' **in** Kirkham, M. (ed.) (1996) *Supervision of Midwives*, Hale: Books for Midwives Press.

Kirkham, M. (ed.) (1996) *Supervision of Midwives*, Hale: Books for Midwives Press.

Kirkham, M.J. and Perkins, E.R. (eds) (1997) *Reflections on Midwifery*, London: Baillière Tindall.

Kirkman, S. (1994) 'Diploma in midwifery to honours degree and beyond', *Midwives Chronicle and Nursing Notes*, 107: 326–327.

Kitzinger, J. (1990) 'Strategies of the Early Childbirth Movement: a case-study of the National Childbirth Trust' in Garcia, J., Kilpatrick, R. and Richards, M. (eds) (1990) *The Politics of Maternity Care: Services for Childbearing Women in Twentieth-Century Britain*, Oxford: Clarendon Press.

Kitzinger, S. (1962) *The Experience of Childbirth*, London: Camelot Press.

——(1979) *The Good Birth Guide*, Glasgow: Fontana Paperbacks.

——(1987) *Freedom and Choice in Childbirth: Making Pregnancy and Birth Plans*, Harmondsworth: Penguin.

——(1988) *Freedom and choice in childbirth*, Harmondsworth: Penguin.

——(2000) *Rediscovering Birth*, London: Little, Brown and Company.

——(2002) *Birth Your Way*, London: Dorling Kindersley Limited.

——(2006) *Birth Crisis*, London: Routledge.

Kitzinger, S. and Davis, J.A. (eds) (1978) *The Place of Birth*, Oxford: Oxford University Press.

Kitzinger, S. and Simkin, P. (eds) (1986) *Episiotomy and the Second Stage of Labor*, Seattle: Pennypress Inc.

Klein, R. (1995) *The New Politics of the NHS*, 3rd edn, London: Longman.

Koven, S. and Michel, S. (1990) 'Womanly duties, maternalist politics, and the origins of welfare states in France, Germany, Great Britain, and the United States, 1880–1920', *American History Review*, 95, 1076–108.

Koven, S. and Michel, S. (eds) (1993) *Mothers of a New World: Maternalist Politics and the Origins of Welfare States*, London: Routledge.

Ladd-Taylor, M. (1988) '"Grannies" and "Spinsters": Midwife education under the Sheppard-Towner Act', *Journal of Social History*, 22, 255–75.

——(1993) '"My work came out of agony and grief": Mothers and the making of the Sheppard-Towner Act' in Koven, S. and Michel, S. (eds) (1993) *Mothers of a New World: Maternalist Politics and the Origins of Welfare States*, London: Routledge, 321–42.

Lang, S.F. (2007) 'Maternal mortality and the State in British India, c.1840–c.1920', unpublished thesis, Anglia Ruskin University.

Larson, M.S. (1977) *The Rise of Professionalism: A Sociological Analysis*, Berkeley: University of California Press.

Leak, W.N. (1952) 'Social trends and home confinements', *British Medical Journal*, 1, 435.

Leap, N. and Hunter, B. (1993) *The Midwife's Tale: An Oral History From Handywoman to Professional Midwife*, London: Scarlet Press.

Leathard, A. (1990) *Healthcare provision: past, present and future*, London: Chapman & Hall.

Leavitt, J.W. (ed.) (1984) *Women and Health in America: Historical Readings*, Wisconsin: University of Wisconsin Press.

——(1984) 'Birthing and anaesthesia: the debate over Twilight Sleep' in Leavitt, J.W. (ed.) (1984) *Women and Health in America: Historical Readings*, Wisconsin: University of Wisconsin Press.

——(1986) *Brought to Bed: Childbearing in America, 1750–1950*, Oxford: Oxford University Press.

——(2009) *Make Room for Daddy: The Journey from Waiting Room to Birthing Room*, Chapel Hill: The University of North Carolina Press.

Leavitt, J.W. and Walton, W. (1984) '"Down to death's door": Women's perception of childbirth in America', in Leavitt, J.W. (ed.) (1984) *Women and Health in America: Historical Readings*, Wisconsin: University of Wisconsin Press.

Lee, G. (1997) 'The concept of "continuity" – What does it mean?' in Kirkham, M.J. and Perkins, E.R. (eds) (1997) *Reflections on Midwifery*, London: Baillière Tindall.

Lewis, J. (1980) *The Politics of Motherhood: Child and Maternal Welfare in England, 1900–1939*, London: McGill-Queens University Press.

——(1986) *What Price Community Medicine? The Philosophy, Practice and Politics of Public Health since 1919*, Brighton: Prentice-Hall.

——(1995) 'Family provision of health and welfare in the mixed economy of care in the late nineteenth and twentieth centuries', *Social History of Medicine*, 8, 1–16.

LGB (1892) *Report from the select committee on midwifery registration*.

——(1909) *Report of the Departmental Committee to Consider the Working of the Midwives Act 1902*, volumes 1 & 2, xxxiii, cd 4822.

——(1914–16) 'Maternal mortality in connection with childbearing and its relation to infant mortality', *LGB 43th Annual Report, 1914–15 Supplement*, xxv, cd 8055.

——(1917) 'Maternal mortality', *44th Annual report of the LGB, 1914–16* cd 8085.

Llewelyn Davies, M. (ed) (1915, reprinted 1978) *Maternity: Letters from Working Women collected by the Women's Co-operative Guild*, London: Virago.

——(ed.) (1931, reprinted 1990) *Life As We Have Known It By Co-operative Working Women*, London: Virago.

Logan, D.D. and MacKenzie, E.K. (1945) 'Domiciliary midwifery and the family doctor', *British Medical Journal*, 2, 294–96.

Løkke, A. (1997) 'The "Antiseptic" Transformation of Danish Midwives, 1860–1920', **in** Marland, H. and Rafferty, A.M. (eds) (1997) *Midwives, Society and Childbirth: Debates and Controversies in the Modern Period, London: Routledge*.

Loudon, I. (1984) 'The concept of the family doctor', *Bulletin of the History Medicine*, 58(3), 347–62.

——(1986) *Medical Care and the General Practitioner, 1730–1850*, Oxford: Clarendon Press.

——(1986) 'Obstetric care, social class, and maternal mortality', *British Medical Journal*, 293, 606–8.

——(1986) 'Deaths in childbed', *Medical History*, 30, 1–41.

——(1987) 'Puerperal fever, the Streptococcus, and Sulphonamides, 1911–45', *British Medical Journal*, 295, 485–90.

——(1990) 'Obstetrics and the General Practitioner', *British Medical Journal*, ii, 703–7.

——(1992) *Death in Childbirth: An International Study of Maternal Care and Maternal Mortality, 1800–1950*, Oxford: Clarendon Press.

——(2008) 'General practitioners and obstetrics: a brief history', *Journal of the Royal Society of Medicine*, 101(11) 531–35.

Loudon, I. (ed.) (1995) *Childbed Fever: A Documentary History*, London: Routledge.

Macfarlane, A.J. (1979) 'Variations in numbers of births and perinatal mortality by day of the week', *British Medical Journal*, i, 750–51.

Macfarlane, A., Mugford, M., Henderson, J., Furtado, A., Stevens, J. and Dunn, A. (2000) *Birth Counts: Statistics of Pregnancy and Childbirth, Volume 2 – Tables*, London: The Stationary Office.

Mander, R. (1983) 'Stop and consider: student midwife wastage in training', *Research and the Midwife Conference Proceedings*.

Marks, L.V. (1994) *Model Mothers: Jewish Mothers and Maternity Provision in East London, 1870–1939*, Oxford: Clarendon Press.

——(1995) '"They're magicians". Midwives, doctors and hospitals: women's experience of childbirth in East London and Woolwich in the inter-war years', *Oral History*, 23, 46–53.

——(1996) *Metropolitan Maternity: Maternal and Infant Welfare Services in Early Twentieth Century London*, Amsterdam: Editions Rodopi B.V.

Marland, H. (1993) 'A pioneer in infant welfare: the Huddersfield scheme, 1903–20', *Social History of Medicine*, 6, 25–50.

——(1995) 'Questions of competence: the midwife debate in the Netherlands in the early twentieth century', *Medical History*, 39, 317–37.

——(1997) *The Midwife as Health Missionary: The Reform of Dutch Childbirth Practices in the Early Twentieth Century*, **in** Marland, H. and Rafferty, A.M. (eds) (1997) *Midwives, Society and Childbirth: Debates and Controversies in the Modern Period*, London: Routledge.

Marland, H. (ed.) (1993) *The Art of Midwifery: Early Modern Midwives in Europe*, London: Routledge.

Marland, H. and Rafferty, A.M. (eds) (1997) *Midwives, Society and Childbirth: Debates and Controversies in the Modern Period*, London: Routledge.

Mason, V. (1989) *Women's Experience of Maternity Care – A Survey Manual*, London: HMSO.

Mathers, H. and McIntosh, T. (2000) *Born in Sheffield: A History of the Women's Health Services, 1864–2000*, Barnsley: Wharncliffe Books.

Maurice, J.F. (1902) 'Where to get Men', *Contemporary Review*, 81, 79–86.

McAleese, S. (2000) 'Caesarean section for maternal choice?', *Midwifery Matters*, Issue 84.

McCleary, G.F. (1935) *The Maternity and Child Welfare Movement*, London: King.

McGann, S. (1997) 'Archival sources for research into the history of nursing', *Nurse Researcher*, 5(2), 19–29.

McIntosh, J. (1989) 'Models of childbirth and social class: a study of 80 working class primigravidae', **in** Robinson, S. and Thomson, A.M. (eds) (1989) *Midwives, Research and Childbirth: Volume 1*, London: Chapman and Hall.

McIntosh, T. (1997) '"A Price Must be Paid for Motherhood": The Experience of Maternity in Sheffield, 1879–1939', unpublished thesis, University of Sheffield.

——(1998) 'Profession, skill or domestic duty? Midwifery in Sheffield, 1881–1936', *Social History of Medicine*, 11(3), 403–20.

——(2000) '"An abortionist city": Maternal mortality, abortion, and birth control in Sheffield, 1920–40', *Medical History*, 44, 75–96.

——(2010) 'Exploring the history of birth: a case study of midwifery care in 1930s England', *MIDIRS*, 20(2), 159–63.

——(2010) 'Using historical research to make sense of our past, present and future. Part 1: Why explore history?', *The Practising Midwife*, 13(11), 34–35.

——(2011) 'Using historical research to make sense of our past, present and future. Part 2: Uncovering source material', *The Practising Midwife*, 14(2), 27–29.

——(2011) 'Using historical research to make sense of our past, present and future. Part 3: Finding and using historical sources', *The Practising Midwife*, 14(4), 37–38.

——(2011) 'Using historical research to make sense of our past, present and future. Part 4: History in context and disseminating findings', *The Practising Midwife*, 14(7), 35–36.

——(2011) 'Direct maternal deaths due to puerperal fever: Back to the future', *British Journal of Midwifery*, 19(4), 212–14.

McLaren, A. (1999) *Twentieth-century Sexuality: A History*, Oxford: Blackwell Publishers Ltd.

Mechling, J. (1975) 'Advice to historians on advice to mothers', *Journal of Social History*, 9, 44–63.

Methven, R.C. (1982) 'The antenatal booking interview: recording an obstetric history or relating with a mother to be?', *Research and the Midwife Conference Proceedings 1982*, 63–95.

Mein-Smith, P. (1986) *Maternity in Dispute: New Zealand 1920–1939*, Wellington: New Zealand Government.

Michael, A.M. (1952) 'Hypnosis in childbirth', *British Medical Journal*, 1, 734.

Miller Wood, L. and Camps, F.E. (1937) 'Puerperal infections in relation to midwifery attendance', *British Medical Journal*, ii, 811–12.

Ministry of Health (1932) *Final Report of the Departmental Committee on Maternal Mortality and Morbidity*.

Mitchell, J. and Oakley, A. (1976) *The Rights and Wrongs of Women*, Harmondsworth: Penguin.

——(1937) *Report on an Investigation into Maternal Mortality*, xi, cmd 5422.

Moir, D.D. (1980) *Obstetric Anaesthesia and Analgesia*, London: Baillière Tindall.

Moorhead, J. (1996) *New Generations: 40 Years of Birth in Britain*, London: HMSO.

Morris, N. (1960) 'Human relations in obstetric practice', *The Lancet*, i: 7130.

Moscucci, O. (1993) *The Science of Woman: Gynaecology and Gender in England, 1800–1929*, Cambridge: Cambridge University Press.

Mottram, J. (1997) *State Control in Local Context: Public Health and Midwife Regulation in Manchester, 1900–1914* in Marland, H. and Rafferty, A.M. (eds) (1997) *Midwives, Society and Childbirth: Debates and Controversies in the Modern Period*, London: Routledge.

Mugford, A. and Macfarlane, A. (2000) *Birth counts: statistics of pregnancy and childbirth*, London: The Stationary Office.

Munro Kerr, J.M. (1933) *Maternal Mortality and Morbidity: A Study of Their Problems*, Edinburgh: E. & S. Livingstone Ltd.

Munro Kerr, J.M., Johnstone, R.W. and Phillips, M.H. (eds) (1954) *Historical Review of British Obstetrics and Gynaecology 1800–1950*, London: E. & S. Livingstone Ltd.

Murphy-Lawless, J. (1998) *Reading Birth and Death: A History of Obstetric Thinking*, Cork: Cork University Press.

Myles, M.F. (1961) *A Textbook for Midwives*, 4th edn, Edinburgh: E. & S. Livingstone Ltd.

——(1968) *A Textbook for Midwives*, 6th edn, Edinburgh: E. & S. Livingstone Ltd.

——(1975) *Textbook for Midwives: with Modern Concepts of Obstetric and Neonatal Care*, 8th edn, Edinburgh: Churchill Livingstone.

NCT (1996) 'Midwife caseloads: an NCT policy statement', *Midwifery Matters*, Issue 71.

Nelson, M.K. (1983) 'Working class women, middle class women and models of childbirth', *Social Problems*, 30(3), 284–97.

Newman, G. (1906) *Infant Mortality: A Social Problem*, London.

Newsholme, A. (1935) *Fifty Years in Public Health*, London: Allen & Unwin.

——(1936) *The Last Thirty Years in Public Health*, London: Allen & Unwin.

Nicol, A. and Sheppard, J. (1985) 'Why keep hospital clinical records?', *British Medical Journal*, 290, 263–64.

NMC (2004) *Midwives Rules and Standards*, London: NMC.

Oakley, A. (1976) 'Wise woman and medicine man: changes in the management of childbirth' **in** Mitchell, J. and Oakley, A. (1976) *The Rights and Wrongs of Women*, Harmondsworth: Penguin Books.

——(1980) *Women Confined: Towards a Sociology of Childbirth*, Oxford: Martin Robertson.

——(1981) *From Here to Maternity: Becoming a Mother*, Harmondsworth: Pelican Books.

——(1981) 'Interviewing women: a contradiction in terms' **in** Roberts, H. (ed.) (1981) *Doing Feminist Research*, London: Routledge and Kegan Paul.

——(1984) *The Captured Womb: a History of the Medical Care of Pregnant Women*, London: Wiley-Blackwell.

——(1986) 'The history of ultrasonography in obstetrics', *Birth* 13, 8–13.

O'Driscoll, K., Stronge, J.M. and Minogue, M. (1973) 'Active Management of Labour' *British Medical Journal*, 3, 135–37.

O'Driscoll, K. and Meagher, D. (1980) *Active Management of Labour*, London: W.B. Saunders Company Ltd.

ley, W.H.F. (1934) 'Prevention of puerperal sepsis in general practice', *British Medical Journal*, i, 1017–19.

Page, L.A. (1992) 'Choice, control and continuity: the 3 "Cs"', *Modern Midwife*, July/August, 8–10.

Page, L.A. (ed.) (1995) *Effective Group Practice in Midwifery: Working with Women*, Oxford: Blackwell Scientific.

Paine, C.G. (1931) 'The source of infection in a minor outbreak of puerperal fever', *British Medical Journal*, i, 1082–83.

Pantin, C.G. (1996) 'A study of maternal mortality and midwifery on the Isle of Man, 1882–1961', *Medical History*, 40, 141–72.

Paranjothy, S. and Thomas, J. (2001) *Royal College of Obstetricians and Gynaecologists Clinical Effectiveness Support Unit. National Sentinel Ceasarean Section Audit Report*, London: RCOG Press.

Peretz, E. (1990) 'A maternity service for England and Wales: Local authority maternity care in the inter-war period in Oxfordshire and Tottenham' **in** Garcia, J., Kilpatrick, R. and Richards, M. (eds) (1990) *The Politics of Maternity Care: Services for Childbearing Women in Twentieth-Century Britain*, Oxford: Clarendon Press.

——(1992) 'Maternal and Child Welfare in England and Wales Between the Wars: A Comparative Regional Study', unpublished thesis, Middlesex University.

Perkins, E.R. (1991) 'What do women want? Asking consumers' views', *Midwives Chronicle*, 104, 347–54.

Perkins, E.R. and Unell, J. (1997) 'Continuity and choice in practice: a study of a community-based team midwifery scheme' **in** Kirkham, M.J. and Perkins, E.R. (eds) (1997) *Reflections on Midwifery*, London: Baillière Tindall.

Perks, R. and Thomson, A. (eds) (2006) *The Oral History Reader*, 2nd edn, Abingdon: Routledge.

Phillips, A. and Rakusen, J. (eds) (1978) *Our Bodies Ourselves: A Health Book By and For Women*, Harmondsworth: Penguin Books Ltd.

Phillips, M. (1935) 'Maternal care', *The Lancet*, ii, 1107–9.

Philpott, R.H. (1972) 'Graphic records in labour', *British Medical Journal*, 4, 163.

Phoenix, A. (1990) 'Black women and the maternity services' **in** Garcia, J., Kilpatrick, R. and Richards, M. (eds) (1990) *The Politics of Maternity Care: Services for Childbearing Women in Twentieth-Century Britain*, Oxford: Clarendon Press.

Pitcock, C.D.H. and Clark, R.B. (1992) 'From Fanny to Fernand: the developments of consumerism in pain control during the birth process', *American Journal of Obstetrics and Gynaecology*, 167, 581–87.

Porter, R. (1997) *The Greatest Benefit to Mankind: A Medical History of Humanity from Antiquity to the Present*, London: HarperCollins Publishers.

Priya, J. (1992) *Birth traditions*, Shaftesbury: Element Books.

Radcliffe, W. (1947) *The secret instrument*, London: Heinemann.

——(1967) *Milestones in midwifery*, Bristol: J Wright.

Radford, N. and Thompson, A. (1988) *Direct Entry: A Preparation for Midwifery Practice*, Guildford: University of Surrey.

Radford, T. (1880) *Observations on the caesarean section*, London: J&A Churchill.

RCOG (1948) *Maternity in Great Britain: A Survey of Social and Economic Aspects of Pregnancy and Childbirth undertaken by a Joint Committee of the Royal College of Obstetricians and Gynaecologists and the Population Investigation Committee*, London: Oxford University Press.

Reagan, J.L. (1995) 'Linking midwives and abortion in the progressive era', *Bulletin of the History of Medicine*, 69:569–598.

Reid, L. (2011) *Midwifery in Scotland: A History*, Edinburgh: Scottish History Press.

Rhodes, M. (1999) '"You worked on your own, making your own decisions and coping on your own": Midwifery knowledge, practice and independence in the workplace in Britain, 1936 to the early 1950's', *Dynamis*, 19, 191–214.

Roberts, E. (1984) *A Woman's Place: An Oral History of Working Class Women 1890–1940*, London: Wiley-Blackwell.

Roberts, H. (1955) *Analgesia for Midwives*, London: E. & S. Livingstone Ltd.

Roberts, H. (ed.) (1981) *Doing Feminist Research*, London: Routledge and Kegan Paul.

Robertson, J. (1917) 'The child welfare campaign and the position of the medical officer of health', *Public Health*, 30, 2–5.

Robinson, J. (1982) 'The maternity defence fund: complaints confined to childbirth', *Nursing Mirror*, 155(10) 14–15.

Robinson, S. (1980) *Midwifery Manpower*, London: Chelsea College, University of London, Nursing Education Research Unit Occasional Papers.

——(1990) 'Maintaining the independence of the midwifery profession: a continuing struggle,' in Garcia, J., Kilpatrick, R. and Richards, M. (eds) (1990) *The Politics of Maternity Care: Services for Childbearing Women in Twentieth-Century Britain*, Oxford: Clarendon Press.

——(1991) 'Preparation for practice: the educational experiences and career intentions of newly qualified midwives' **in** Robinson, S. and Thomson A. (eds) (1991) *Midwives, research and childbirth*, volume 2, London: Chapman & Hall.

Robinson, S., Golden, J. and Bradley, S. (1981) 'A preliminary report of the research project on the role and responsibilities of the midwife: Part 1', *Midwives Chronicle*, 94, 11–15.

Robinson, S. and Thomson, A.M. (eds) (1989) *Midwives, Research and Childbirth: Volume 1*, London: Chapman and Hall.

——(1991) *Midwives, Research and Childbirth: Volume 2*, London: Chapman and Hall.

——(1991) 'Research and midwifery; moving into the 1990s' **in** Robinson, S. and Thomson, A.M. (eds) (1991) *Midwives, Research and Childbirth: Volume 2*, London: Chapman and Hall.

Romney, M. (1981) 'Pre-delivery shaving: an unjustified assault' **in** *The Role of the Midwife: First Annual Conference, Sheffield, 1981*, London: Association of Radical Midwives.

Roper, W., Logan, W. and Tierney, A. (1990) *The Elements of Nursing Based on a Model of Living*, 3rd edn, London: Churchill Livingstone.

Rowntree, B.S. (1901) *Poverty: A Study of Town Life*, London.

Salzmann, K.D. (1955) 'The nature and some hazards of obstetrics in general practice', *British Medical Journal*, 2, 15.

Sandall, J. (1997) 'Midwives, burnout and continuity of care', *British Journal of Midwifery*, 5(2), 106–11.

Savage, W. (1988) *A Savage Enquiry: Who Controls Childbirth?* London: Virago Press Limited.

Schwarz, E.W. (1990) 'The Engineering of Childbirth: a new obstetric programme as reflected in British obstetric textbooks, 1960–1980.' in Garcia, J., Kilpabrick, R. and Richards, M. (eds) (1990) *The Politics of Maternity Care: Services for Childbearing Women in Twentieth Century Britain*, Oxford: Clarendon Press.

Shorter, E. (1983) *A History of Women's Bodies*, London: Basic Books.

Sklar, K.K. (1990) 'A call for comparisons', *American History Review*, 95, 1109–14.

——(1993) 'The historical foundations of women's power in the creation of the American welfare state, 1830–1930' in Koven, S. and Michel, S. (eds) (1993) *Mothers of a New World: Maternalist Politics and the Origins of Welfare States*, London: Routledge.

Skocpol, T. (1992) *Protecting Soldiers and Mothers: the Politics of Social Provision in the United States, 1870s–1920s*, Cambridge: Belknap Press.

Sleep, J. (1983) 'The West Berkshire episiotomy trial', *Research and the Midwife Conference Proceedings.*

——(1991) 'Perineal care: a *series of five randomized controlled trials'* in Robinson, S. and Thomson, A.M. (eds) (1991) *Midwives, Research and Childbirth: Volume 2*, London: Chapman and Hall.

Sleep, J., Grant, A., Garcia, J., Elbourne, D., Spencer, J. and Chalmers, I. (1984) 'West Berkshire perineal management trial', *British Medical Journal*, 587–590.

Smellie, W. (1752) *A treatise on the theory and practice of midwifery*, London.

Smith, E.M. (1921) 'The role of the maternity hospital in public health work', *Public Health*, 34, 67–72.

Smith, J.F. (1997) *Labour Days: Having a Baby Before the Birth of the National Health Service ...*, Elland: Jay Publishing.

Spring Rice, M. (1939, reprinted 1981) *Working Class Wives: Their Health and Conditions*, London: Virago Press.

Stacey, J.E. (1931) 'Remarks on "failed forceps"', *British Medical Journal*, ii, 1073–78.

Stacey, M., Reid, M., Heath, C. and Dingwall, R. (eds) (1977) *Health and the Division of Labour*, London: Croom Helm.

Stapleton, H. (1997) 'Choice in the face of uncertainty' in Kirkham, M.J. and Perkins, E.R. (eds) (1997) *Reflections on Midwifery*, London: Baillière Tindall.

Steadman Jones, G. (1984) *Outcast London: A Study in the Relationship Between Classes in Victorian Society*, 2nd edn, Oxford: Clarendon Press.

Stock, J. and Wraight, A. (1993) *Developing Continuity of Care in Maternity Services*, Brighton: Institute of Manpower Studies.

Stopes, M. (1918) *Married Love*, London: Fifield & Co.

——(1919) *Wise Parenthood*, London: Fifield and Co.

——(1925) *Radiant Motherhood*, London: G.P. Putnams & Sons Ltd.

Studd, J. (1973) 'Partograms and nomograms of cervical dilatation in management of primigravid labour', *British Medical Journal*, 4, 451–55.

Summers, A. (1989) 'The mysterious demise of Sarah Gamp: The domiciliary nurse and her detractors c. 1830–60', *Victorian Studies*, 32(3), 365–86.

Sweet, B.R. (ed.) (1984) *Mayes' Midwifery: A Textbook for Midwives*, 10th edn, London: Baillière Tindall.

——(1988) *Mayes' Midwifery: A Textbook for Midwives*, 11th edn, London: Baillière Tindall.

——(1997) *Mayes' Midwifery: A Textbook for Midwives*, 12th edn, London: Baillière Tindall.

Sweet, H.M. and Dougall, R. (2008) *Community Nursing and Primary Healthcare in Twentieth-Century Britain*, London: Routledge.

Symon, A. (2006) 'Risk and choice: knowledge and control' in Symon, A. (ed.) (2006) *Risk and Choice in Maternity Care: An international perspective*, Edinburgh: Elsevier.

Symon, A. (ed.) (2006) *Risk and Choice in Maternity Care: An international perspective*, Edinburgh: Elsevier.

Szreter, S. (1996) *Fertility, Class and Gender in Britain, 1860–1940*, Cambridge: Cambridge University Press.

Szreter, S. and Fisher, K. (2010) *Sex Before the Sexual Revolution: Intimate Life in England 1918–1963*, Cambridge: Cambridge University Press.

Tacchi, D. (1971) 'Towards easier childbirth', *The Lancet*, ii, 1134–36.

Tansey, E.M. and Christie, D.A. (eds) (2000) *Looking at the Unborn: Historical Aspects of Obstetric Ultrasound*, Wellcome Witnesses to Twentieth Century Medicine, London: The Wellcome Trust.

Tew, M. (1995) *Safer Childbirth? A Critical History of Maternity Care*, 2nd edn, London: Nelson Thornes.

Thane, P. (1991) 'Visions of gender in the British welfare state' in Bock, G. and Thane, P. (eds) (1991) *Maternity and Gender Policies: Women and the Rise of European Welfare States, 1880s–1950s*, London: Routledge.

Thom, D. (1998) *Nice Girls and Rude Girls: Women Workers in World War I*, London: I.B. Tauris.

Thomas, P. (1996) *Every Woman's BirthRights*, London: Thorsons.

——(1998) *Every Birth is Different: Women's Experiences in Their Own Words*, London: Headline Book Publishing.

Thomas, L.M. (2003) *Politics of the womb: women, reproduction and the State in Kenya*, Berkley: University of California Press.

Thompson, A. (1997) *Establishing the Scope of Practice: Organizing European Midwifery in the Inter-War Years 1919–1938* in Marland, H. and Rafferty, A.M. (eds) (1997) *Midwives, Society and Childbirth: Debates and Controversies in the Modern Period*, London: Routledge.

——(1984) 'Antenatal care: An examination of the midwife's contribution', *Research and the Midwife Conference Proceedings 1984*, 135–63.

Thompson, A. and Robinson, S. (1985) 'Dissemination of midwifery research and how this has been facilitated in the UK', *Midwifery*, 1, 52–53.

Thompson, E.P. (1967) 'Time, work-discipline and industrial capitalism', *Past and Present*, 38(1), 56–97.

Titmuss, R.M. (1950) *Problems of social policy*, London: HMSO.

Topping, A. (1936) 'Maternal mortality and public opinion', *Public Health*, 49, 342–9.

Towler, J. and Bramall, J. (1986) *Midwives in History and Society*, London: Croom Helm Ltd.

Townsend, P., Davidson, N. and Whitehead, M. (1992) *Inequalities in Health: The Black Report and The Health Divide*, London: Penguin Books.

Versluysen, M.C. (1980) 'Old wives' tales? Women healers in English history' in Davies, C. (ed.) (1980) *Re-writing Nursing History*, London: Croom Helm.

Walker, J. (1996) 'BUMPS: birth under midwifery practice scheme', *Midwifery Matters*, Issue 69.

——(1999) 'BUMPS up and running: Changing Childbirth 6 years on', *Midwifery Matters*, Issue 82.

Walsh, D. (2003) 'Risk management is not objective (editorial)', *British Journal of Midwifery*, 11(8), 474.

——(2007) *Evidence-based Care for Normal Labour and Birth: A Guide for Midwives*, Abingdon: Routledge.

Walton, I. and Hamilton, M. (1995) *Midwives and Changing Childbirth*, Hale: Books for Midwives Press Ltd.

Ward, M.E. and Adams, M.E. (1979) 'A masters degree in midwifery', *Midwives Chronicle*, 92, 37–38.

Watts, G. (1997) 'Changing Childbirth?' *Midwifery Matters*, Issue 75.

Webb, J. and Weston-Edwards, P. (1951) 'Recent trends in maternal mortality', *The Medical Officer*, 86, 201–4.

Webster, C. (1982) 'Healthy or hungry thirties?', *History Workshop Journal*, 13, 110–129.

——(1988) *The Health Services Since the War, Volume 1, Problems of Health Care: The National Health Service Before 1957*, London: HMSO.

——(2002) *The National Health Service: A political history*, Oxford: Oxford University Press.

Weisz, G. (2005) *Divide and Conquer: A Comparative History of Medical Specialization*, Oxford: Oxford University Press.

Wertz, R.W. and Wertz, D.C. (1989) *Lying in: A History of Childbirth in America*, 2nd edn, Yale: Yale University Press.

Wesson, N. (1995) *Home Birth: A Practical Guide*, London: Optima.

White, A. (1901) *Efficiency and Empire*, London: Methuen.

Wilkes, J.B. (1992) 'The last of the handywomen', *Midwives Chronicle and Nursing Notes*, 178–79.

Willcocks, A.J. (1967) *The Creation of the National Health Service: A Study of Pressure Groups and a Major Social Policy Decision*, London: Routledge and Kegan Paul.

Williams, A.S. (1997) *Women and Childbirth in the Twentieth Century: A History of the National Birthday Trust Fund 1928–93*, Stroud: Sutton Publishing Limited.

Willocks, J. and Barr, W. (2004) *Ian Donald: A Memoir*, London: RCOG Press.

Wilson, A. (1995) *The Making of Man-Midwifery: Childbirth in England 1660–1770*, London: UCL Press.

Wilson, E. (1977) *Women and the Welfare State*, London: Tavistock.

Winter, J.M. (1979) 'Infant mortality, maternal mortality, and public health in Britain in the 1930s', *Journal of European Economic History*, 8: 439–62.

Witz, A. (1992) *Professions and Patriarchy*, London: Routledge.

Wootton, D. (2007) *Bad Medicine: Doctors Doing Harm Since Hippocrates*, Oxford: Oxford University Press.

Worth, J. (2007) *Call the Midwife*, London: Phoenix.

Wraight, A. (1995) 'Organizational styles and patterns of care' **in** *Continuity of Care to Meet the Challenge of 'Changing Childbirth': Midwifery Educational Resource Pack 3*, London: ENB.

Wraight, A., Ball, J., Secombe, I. and Stock, J. (1993) *Mapping Team Midwifery*, Brighton: Institute of Manpower Studies, University of Sussex.

Young, J. (1928) 'Maternal mortality from puerperal sepsis', *British Medical Journal*, i, 967–71.

——(1950) 'Maternity and The National Health Service', *British Medical Journal*, 1, 392–96.

Yow, V. (2006) '"Do I like them too much?": effects of the oral history interview on the interviewer and vice-versa', **in** Perks, R. and Thomson, A. (eds) (2006) *The Oral History Reader*, 2nd edn, Abingdon: Routledge.

Zander, L. and Chamberlain, G. (eds) (1984) *Pregnancy Care for the 1980s: Based on a Conference Held at the Royal Society of Medicine*, London: The Royal Society of Medicine and Macmillan Press Ltd.

Index